—MAKING—
NATURAL
COSMETICS

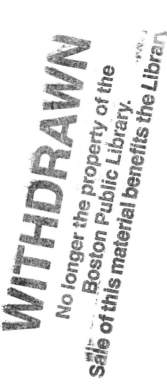

—MAKING—
NATURAL
COSMETICS
BEAUTY THE WAY NATURE INTENDED

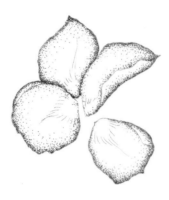

MARGARET BRIGGS

HERMES
HOUSE

This edition is published by Hermes House, an imprint of
Anness Publishing Ltd, Hermes House, 88–89 Blackfriars Road,
London SE1 8HA; tel. 020 7401 2077; fax 020 7633 9499

www.hermeshouse.com; www.annesspublishing.com

Anness Publishing has a new picture agency outlet for images for
publishing, promotions or advertising. Please visit our website
www.practicalpictures.com for more information.

Produced by Omnipress Limited, UK

ETHICAL TRADING POLICY

At Anness Publishing we believe that business should be
conducted in an ethical and ecologically sustainable way, with
respect for the environment and a proper regard to the
replacement of the natural resources we employ.
As a publisher, we use a lot of wood pulp to make high-quality
paper for printing, and that wood commonly comes from spruce
trees. We are therefore currently growing more than 750,000
trees in three Scottish forest plantations. The forests we manage
contain more than 3.5 times the number of trees employed each
year in making paper for the books we manufacture.
Because of this ongoing ecological investment programme, you,
as our customer, can have the pleasure and reassurance of
knowing that a tree is being cultivated on your behalf to naturally
replace the materials used to make the book you are holding.
For further information, go to www.annesspublishing.com/trees

A CIP catalogue record for this book is available from
the British Library.

Previously published as *Natural Cosmetics*

PUBLISHER'S NOTE

Although the advice and information in this book are believed to
be accurate and true at the time of going to press, neither the
author nor the publisher can accept any legal responsibility or
liability for any errors or omissions that may be made nor for any
inaccuracies nor for any harm or injury that comes about from
following instructions or advice in this book.

CONTENTS

  Acacia • Aloe Vera • Almond • Amla • Apricot •
  Arrowroot • Avocado • Basil • Beeswax • Bergamot
  • Bicarbonate of soda • Calendula • Camphor •
  Carob • Carnauba • Centella • Chamomile/Babuna
  • Cinnamon • Citrus oils • Cocoa butter • Cocoa
  powder • Cornflour • Cucumber • *Eclipta alba* •
  Egg • Elder • Evening primrose • Fennel •
  Frankincense • Fuller's earth • Ginger • Gingko •
  Glycerine • Grape seed oil • Groundnut oil • Hemp
  seed oil • Henna • Hibiscus • Horse chestnut
  extract • Honey • Indigo • Jasmine • Jojoba oil •
  Kohl • Lady's mantle • Lanolin • Lavender •
  Lemons • Macadamia nut oil • Myrrh • Neem
  tree/Margosa tree • Nettle • Oats • Olive oil •
  Orange • Palmarosa oil • Patchouli • Peanut oil •
  Petroleum jelly • Propolis • Pumpkin seed oil •
  Rice bran wax • Rosemary • Rose oil • Rose-water
  • Royal jelly • Safflower oil • Sea buckthorn oil •
  Sea salt • Sesame oil • Shea butter • Shilajit •
  Soapberry, soapnut • Spearmint • Sunflower oil •
  Talcum powder • Tamanu oil • Thanaka • Tea tree
  oil • Turmeric • Vetiver • Violet • Vinegar • Walnut
  • Wheat germ oil • Witch hazel • Woad •
  Ylang-ylang • Zinc oxide

INTRODUCTION

WHAT ARE NATURAL COSMETICS?

'My lover is to me a cluster of henna blossoms from the vineyards of En Gedi'

SONG OF SONGS, 1:14

Some people may equate all cosmetics with making us look like something we are not. Well, there's nothing new in that idea, because civilisations have been enhancing their appearance with plants, extracts and minerals for thousands of years. The idea of natural cosmetics today may conjure up an array of commercial products used for the purposes of cleansing, beautifying or altering one's appearance or promoting attractiveness. Cosmetics are basically substances used to enhance or protect the appearance of the body, or to cover up body odour. Cosmetics include skin-care creams, powders and perfumes, as well as lipsticks, nail polishes, eye and facial make-up. Others might include permanent waves or 'perms', hair colours, deodorants, bath oils and bubble baths. Cosmetics can be more than that, in that they can correct deficiencies of the skin or cover up what might be considered flaws or defects. In so doing they can improve self esteem, enhance mood and generally make us feel better. Who hasn't been seduced by the odd lipstick or eye shadow by advertising now and then, when feeling a bit down in the dumps?

Cosmetics, like beauty, are only skin deep, but they can really make a difference. Never mind the fact that you may be sleep deprived, hung over or ill: a bit of 'slap' can give the appearance of health and happiness. Immersing yourself in a fragrant bath for ten minutes can be a real boost.

I've never been one to use a lot of make-up, because I've never had the time or inclination to put it all on. Given the choice of staying in bed for an extra half an hour in the mornings or looking flawless is a complete no brainer as far as I'm concerned, but that doesn't mean that I never use any cosmetics. When you wear a lot of make-up, it becomes a daily chore that has to continue forever. I do try to stick to natural products whenever possible, in the same way that I try to get enough exercise and sleep and eat a healthy diet. Those are the things that will really make a difference to the quality of your skin.

This book is about how you can use natural products, everyday plants and foods to make your own cosmetics. It is a collection of ideas rather than a beauty regime, from which you can pick and choose and adopt or reject. Some of the ideas are current while others have been around for centuries. I just offer them from personal interest and research.

The recipes have been kept simple in most cases and can be made quite cheaply from plants and readily available materials. Exceptions will be in the area of essential oils and some specific ingredients, although a few bottles of essential oils will keep you going for ages. Enjoy!

A SHORT HISTORY OF NATURAL COSMETICS

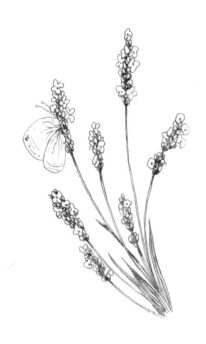

A SHORT HISTORY
OF NATURAL COSMETICS

'A woman without paint is like food without salt.'

ROMAN PLAYWRIGHT, PLAUTUS, C.250–184 BC

Well, there's a statement to get the ball rolling. I
wonder if there was any irony hidden in the line.
Nowadays, in post-feminist times there's quite a lot
to argue with there. We might take offence at either
suggestion, but the salt issue has already been dealt
with in another book. Still, the cosmetics industry is
certainly not down to modern science and technology.
There's a whole list of reasons why people want to
change their looks. Men and women have been
changing their appearance by applying creams, oils
and colouring from minerals for thousands of years.
There is archaeological evidence dating back 6,000
years, to suggest that the ancient Egyptians used
cosmetics and it seems that nearly every civilisation
known since then has used them in one form or other.
The ingredients may have changed a lot, but the
intention remains the same: to enhance physical
appearance and to improve the air around by covering
up or banishing unpleasant odours. Cosmetics became
part of daily life for the Egyptians, hygiene and
health being high on the agenda as well as the
spiritual element attached to wearing make-up.

EGYPTIAN COSMETICS

The early use of cosmetics by the ancient Egyptians seems to have been associated with religious ceremony. It has even been suggested that scented oil may have been used to clean and soften the skin round about 10,000 BC, perhaps by burning resins to make incense. How can anyone tell when it all began? From about 7000 BC olive oil, sesame oil and animal fats appear to have been mixed with scented plants for use in ceremonies and for personal use. By the time the Egyptians began recording events on stone and tablets there was quite a demand for imported myrrh, the resin derived from thorny desert trees in modern Ethiopia, Yemen and Somalia.

The Egyptians believed that everything had a spiritual meaning and application. Perfumes made the body function perfectly. Ra, the sun god, was responsible for all sense of smell and only perfectly perfumed people would be received by the gods when they died.

Cedar oil was the most sacred of oils and the main one used in mummification. Priests believed that certain perfumes could enhance personal power, so they kept their knowledge secret from neighbouring civilisations.

The most famous Egyptian fragrance, called kyphi, was said to induce hypnotic states. In Heliopolis, the city of the sun god and now a suburb of Cairo, priests burnt resins in the morning, myrrh at noon and kyphi at sunset.

ESSENTIAL SKIN OILS

People used oils and creams to protect their skin from the intense sun and drying, sand laden winds. Soft, supple skin prevented cracking, thus keeping the skin healthier and free from infection. Oils and ointments therefore became quite important as a part of regular payment, and trouble brewed when these essentials were withheld during the time of Rameses III, circa 1180 BC.

Herbs such as thyme, chamomile, marjoram and rosemary were used as ingredients, along with scented flowers such as lavender, roses and lilies, in religious ceremonies as well as for embalming. The Egyptians were known to have used natron for this latter purpose.

DEAD GORGEOUS

The ancient Egyptians appreciated beauty so much they protected and preserved it even after death, by mummification. A major substance in this process was natron, a white crystalline mixture of sodium bicarbonate, sodium carbonate, sodium chloride and sodium sulphate. It was mined from dry lake beds and from the banks of the River Nile. The area of Wadi-el-Natrun lies 23 metres (75 feet) below sea level and gets its name from the natron. Known to be mildly antiseptic as well as a good exfoliant and drying substance, it was, all in all, a perfect base for adding oils and fragrances used to preserve the dead. The fragrances exemplified spirituality and beauty and served to cover up the foul odours of decaying flesh, which conjured up or summoned particular deities. So you not only had to look good but also had to smell divine, even in the intense heat of Egypt, without refrigeration or air-conditioning.

The ancient Egyptians recognised that cleanliness was of the utmost importance in the living as well as the dead. To repel body odour men and women were advised to rub seeds of ground carob into the skin, or to place little balls of incense where limbs met. Carob is still used today in some cosmetics.

Natron was the supreme, holistic cleaning product and was used in a variety of ways for personal hygiene and household cleaning. To ensure you were really clean and pure, you needed to smell clean and not give off bad odours that might summon up evil forces.

The closest you can get today to natron is a packet or tub of commercially produced bicarbonate of soda. So many of the age old remedies and applications of bicarbonate of soda can be traced back, like so many other seemingly modern remedies, to the knowledge possessed by the ancient Egyptians. You can read about using modern bicarbonate of soda in later sections.

PEARLY WHITES

As ancient toothpaste, natron could be mixed with a few drops of water to create a paste. A few drops of myrrh could also be added. Myrrh was much prized by the Egyptians as a perfume, incense and healer, and they believed that, when it was added to the toothpaste, it served as a gum protector and improver of oral hygiene.

There is no evidence of toothbrushes, but later Egyptians used a natural brush-cum-toothpaste, miswak, from a tree native to southern Egypt and the Sudan. The twigs from the arak or peelu tree have been used for dental care for centuries.

To improve on their breath the Egyptians also chewed herbs or gargled with milk, despite the fact that milk doesn't spring to mind as the most natural breath freshener.

Red natron was probably tinted by an iron compound in the earth where the natron was extracted.

CONE HEADS

A variety of oils and fats were available for perfumes. One popular basic oil was called balanos, but the lower classes used castor oil. Three techniques for extracting scents were employed. The first was to soak flowers in layers of fat. Creams and pomades were created in this manner. A cone-shaped pomade was worn on top of the head. As the cone melted, scented oil would run down the face and neck. Cones were renewed when necessary. It all sounds a bit messy to me.

The second process, maceration, involved dipping flowers, herbs or fruits into fats or oils and heating them to 65°C (149°F). The mixture was sieved and allowed to cool then shaped into cones or balls. The third, less popular process was to press the essence from flowers or seeds like the wine maker pressing fruit.

KOHL BLACK EYES

Eye make-up is probably the most well known of the Egyptian cosmetics. Both men and women used eye make-up. Although cosmetics in ancient Egypt were certainly used for beautifying, eye make-up served other purposes as well. It had spiritual and medicinal connotations. The popular colours were green and black. Green was originally made from malachite, an oxide of copper. In early times it was applied from the eyebrow to the base of the nose. Later, green eye paint was used for the brows and the corners of the eyes, and eventually the green was replaced with black. This was kohl, usually made of a sulphide of lead called galena.

Putting lead on your face doesn't really seem a good idea nowadays of course, but the Egyptians didn't realise that lead was poisonous. However, galena is said to have had disinfectant properties and to keep the flies away. Mothers would apply kohl to their children's eyes soon after birth to strengthen the eyes to protect from evil. There may also be some protection given from intense sunlight, but I still don't recommend going to your nearest former lead mines or crushing areas and collecting your own!

The malachite came from mines in Sinai where Hathor, the goddess of beauty, love and women, held sway. Galena came from the Red Sea Coast and was given by nomads to the pharaoh. It had to be made into a powder and then mixed with some sort of oily animal fat to make it stick to the areas around the eyes. The palettes, grinders and objects used to apply the make-up have been found in burial sites, showing that kohl was an essential item for the afterlife, even among the humblest of subjects. I wonder if there's any change today, given the huge range of products and prices among leading make up and beauty concerns.

Wealth was displayed by the quality of the containers and applicators used. A burial site discovered at Saqqara exposed fragments of a salve chest with thirty compartments for unguents and oil jars. Around 1400 BC three women were buried with some pretty impressive and costly cosmetics. Two jars contained a cleansing cream made of oil and lime. Lime isn't considered a good substance to have on the skin these days. I wonder what they died from.

Kohl today is mostly made from harmless ingredients. Instead of galena, carbon or charcoal is used, along with plant oils. Soot from burning nuts and seeds and gum resins are often added to the powder. Kohl describes colour rather than ingredients. If you are in Egypt or India, where some home-made kohl is still sold, verify that the product is lead-free before using it. It makes my eyes water just thinking about all that lead.

Kohl is used predominantly by women in the Middle East, North and sub-Saharan Africa and Southern Asia. Men use it to a much lesser extent. Real kohl is sold in a small box with a stick for application. The stick should have a slightly rounded end, like a wooden cotton bud. The traditional way of applying it sounds a little hazardous, given the stick/eye proximity, but I'm told you soon get the hang of it. Actually it doesn't sound that far removed from the old cake eye liner of my youth, except for the small paintbrush instead of the stick. All you needed was a bit of spit and you were away. You're supposed to close the eyes and draw the dampened stick lightly along the lids to leave a smudgy line. Two black eyes? No trouble. Thank goodness for modern kohl pencils.

Made-up eyes were thought to protect the wearer from evil. Making an outline round the eyes thus protected the skin in the same way as an amulet or talisman might be worn. Eyebrows were coloured black for emphasis.

Later the Egyptians crushed up beetle shells to mix with eye paints and create a glittery effect.

LIP COLOURING

Before 4000 BC Egyptians were painting their lips red or blue-black. There was a hierarchy of colours, with only royalty allowed to use red. This may have been red ochre, a sort of clay, mixed with fat or gum resin. Lip gloss, possibly made in the same way, was applied with a brush or spatula. Rouge made from the same ingredients was also used.

MANICURES

Nails were also coloured and no self respecting commander would go into battle without first having a manicure. Again, only royalty could have red nails, with lesser mortals having to make do with paler colours. Manicure sets shaped and conditioned the nails, setting aside the rich and aristocratic from the poorer sections of society.

HENNA

Henna was used to dye greying hair from before 3000 BC. It was also used to paint nails and to decorate the palms of the hands and the soles of feet. Henna powder is still used today in many countries and is associated in India with Lakshmi, the goddess of beauty and good fortune. The elaborate patterns and designs worn on hands to celebrate festivals such as Diwali and Eid have always been a source of fascination to me. When henna is worn it is said to protect the wearer from harm. It was also used to colour fingernails yellow and orange.

HAIR REMOVAL

The Egyptians didn't do facial hair, or any other visible hair (other than men's small moustaches and goatees) and believed it to be a sign of personal neglect and a lack of hygiene. Cleanliness and personal appearance were highly regarded. Priests observed strict cleanliness by washing several times a day and being clean shaven all over, to keep lice away. The eggs of these dear little chaps, ever present in modern times, have been found in the hair of mummies.

Modern soap had not yet been invented, so oil was probably used to soften the skin and hairs of the area to be shaved. Tweezers were used for removing individual facial hairs.

Men and women used razors for removing body hair, as well as creams.

Some other remedies for removing hair from the body are particularly eye watering. To avoid razor burn, how about boiling the bones of a bird and mixing with fly droppings, lard, sycamore milk, gum, cucumber and rock salt, applied warm? Not for you? What about a nice skin renewal treatment to follow, made of honey, red natron and salt? This at least sounds more like some modern treatments. Mixed together, it was rubbed into the limbs.

GREYING HAIR

Some recipes for covering grey hair other than using henna must have resulted from either desperation or a desire to see someone you didn't like suffer for their vanity. The most bizarre, probably the result of a belief in magic, was to use donkey liver that had been left to fester and rot. This was then cooked and added to lard before rubbing into the hair. Another advocates using a cooked mouse, rotted in lard. Ox or calf blood from a black ox was boiled in oil in the hope of transferring colour to greying hair. A preventative treatment suggested making the black horn of a gazelle into an ointment with oil to prevent grey hairs appearing.

The most successful treatment for dyeing the hair would have come from juniper berries and two unknown plants. This was kneaded into a paste with oil and heated. The plant pigment would temporarily dye the hair and the astringent properties of the juniper berries would have stimulated the scalp. If I had been worried about having grey hair, I'd have got a wig instead! Coming from a family whose hair starts turning grey very early, some of us just learn to live with it — or dye it with safer, more reliable methods.

STYLES, CURLS AND WIGS

Common people generally wore their hair short. Young girls kept their hair in plaits while boys had shaved heads with one braided lock worn on one side. Egyptian men shaved their head in order to avoid getting lice.

Elaborate wigs and hairpieces were seemingly quite popular among men and women for special occasions. These were usually made from human hair but sometimes from wool. When not being used they were kept in special boxes. Evidence suggests that cones described above would protect the hair or give the wig a pleasant fragrance.

Wig wearing doesn't mean that people didn't like to

keep their own hair looking good. All manner of paraphernalia has been found including combs, a type of setting lotion made from beeswax and resin, hair pins and a bronze object, thought to be used for curling the hair. Other tools used in the beauty ritual that have been found include short, fine tooth combs, hair pins, and a small bronze implement with a pivoting blade, thought to be a hair curler. Egyptian commanders would curl their hair before embarking on a spot of killing in times of war. You had to look your best, even if the worst happened.

BALDNESS

You would think that a society so concerned about hair growing in the wrong places and with wigs available that baldness wouldn't have been an issue, especially when many were shaving their heads anyway to avoid lice and other nasties. Chopped lettuce was placed on bald patches or the head was treated with oils and fats.

ANTI-AGEING CREAMS

Egyptians didn't live to a ripe old age, but I suppose all that sand, sun and sensual living aged the skin quite a lot. I wonder if skin cancer was a problem. Exposure to intense sun would certainly cause wrinkling and drying. A mixture containing frankincense, oil, grasses and plant juices was mixed with wax to apply as a remedy. Juniper berries were sometimes added, along with other plants that provided colouring. This could also be used to cover scars and burns. Red ochre, kohl and sycamore juice were also used on burns, and honey was a known antibacterial, used to promote healing. Oil from fenugreek seeds is also said to have been used to help condition the skin.

TATTOOS

Tattooing was practised, possibly as early as 4000 BC. Female clay figures dating from this time, decorated with dots, dashes and lines have survived. Mummies of dancers and concubines, from the Middle Kingdom 2040–1640 BC, have geometric designs tattooed on chests, shoulders and arms. From later times, tattoos of the god Bes were found on the thighs and lower pelvic areas of young women. Tattoos were all similar to the blue/black designs seen in North African and Western Asian women.

EYE TREATMENTS

To cool the eyes, jasper or serpentine was finely ground, mixed with water and applied to the lids. Another recipe used ground carob and fermented honey. An eyewash was prepared from ground celery and hemp. In-growing eyelashes seemed to be a problem of the times.

MAKE-UP BOXES

A rouge consisting of red ochre and fat, possibly with a little added resin, has survived for 4,000 years. That's quite a shelf life. Make-up was stored in jars that were kept in special boxes. Perhaps as a forerunner to the handbag, women carried their make-up boxes to parties with them. Men also wore make-up, but left their supplies at home.

WASHING

Most Egyptians washed daily in the river or from a basin at home. Public bathhouses have been excavated at Tebtunis, the oldest dating to around

300 BC. There were showers, stone basins and a system to heat water. Better-off Egyptians had wooden or clay footbaths for washing their feet. Wealthy homes also had a room and servants to pour jugs of water over their masters. They had washbasins and probably filled them with a natron and salt solution from jugs. Sand was perhaps used as a scouring agent. Some basins even had pipes to drain the water away. People rubbed themselves daily with a perfumed, soothing oil that had soaked in scented wood. The mixture was left in a pot until the oil absorbed the wood scent.

SOAP

When fats or oils are mixed with a strong alkali the fats are split into fatty acids and glycerine. The sodium or potassium in the alkali joins with the fatty acid as the basis of soap. Spaniards and other Mediterranean people used burnt seaweed to provide the alkali they needed. The most common early soaps were made from potash and pearlash. Early references to the use of soap include the Babylonians, about 2800 BC, and the Phoenicians, around 600 BC. The Egyptians used natron, as described above, mixed with animal and vegetable oils. This was also used to treat skin disease.

Pliny described Roman soap as being made from goat fat and wood ash, with salt added to harden it into bars. Excavations in Pompeii have revealed a soap factory containing bars of soap, but this would have been for washing textiles rather than for personal hygiene. The Romans favoured olive oil, perfumed oils and extracts and sand to clean their bodies, after a good steam. See a later section in this chapter for more on soap.

GREEK AND ROMAN TIMES

In ancient Greek times women advertised their marital status with their hairstyle. During the classical period women wore their hair long, except when they were in mourning. At this time they cut their hair short. Slaves also wore short hair. Before the fifth century women's hair fell over the shoulders and back and was often fastened by a headband. After the fifth century BC there were a greater a number of possibilities and during Hellenistic times hair was artificially waved and curled. Body hair was mostly removed.

As ideas and civilisations rose and fell, people used to paint their faces in a similar way to the Egyptians. Ancient Greek women had access to many substances that they used to improve their health and appearance. Honey was used to moisturise the skin and olive oil was used to protect it. Unlike the Egyptians, the women of ancient Greece did not use tattoos or other symbolic markings on their skin.

Greek women used very little in the way of cosmetics but they used olive oil, lanolin and tallow as a base and charcoal and earth colours for pigments. Ground charcoal could be mixed with olive oil for eye shadow, like kohl. Red pigment could be mixed with beeswax and olive oil for a paste to use on their lips. Unfortunately they used white lead to whiten their skin. Used over time, these chemicals poisoned their bodies. Both Romans and ancient Egyptians used cosmetics containing mercury, which was obviously not a good idea either, with the benefit of hindsight.

The word 'cosmetic' has its roots in Roman times, coming from the Latin *cosmetae*, which was first used to describe female slaves who had the job of bathing their masters in perfume. They spent their days dissolving various ingredients, in their own saliva, as described in one record, and mixing them with spatulas and ring-shaped mixers made of wood, bone, ivory, amber, glass or metal.

The Romans were, it seems, more interested in bathing in fragrance than improving the science or ingredients used in cosmetics. They were also perhaps the most lavish users of aromatic spices. Style over content was the order of the day and vanity ruled. The Egyptian methods were still used and spread throughout the Mediterranean.

The Romans incorporated spices into cosmetics. Even soldiers used perfumes from the East. Wealthy Romans so overindulged themselves in fragrance that an edict forbidding such foolish excess attempted to reduce demand for incense. By the first century AD Romans were burning 2,800 tons of imported frankincense and 550 tons of myrrh per year. Both were more costly than gold.

As a note of interest, this is where the word 'perfume' comes from: *Per*, meaning through and *fumus*, the Latin for 'smoke'. Roman perfumes followed Greek traditions but one of the popular scents appears to have been made by mixing sandalwood or musk with cinnamon, ginger and vanilla.

Balms and oils for use after bathing were popular and the addition of spices thickened them as well as making them more fragrant.

FOUNDATIONS AND MASKS

Women in Roman Britain used a foundation cream made from animal fat, starch and tin oxide. Another concoction, called *biacca*, contained white lead. This was used to cover up imperfections of the skin. It was made from wax, honey and fat and was apparently quite toxic on occasions. Roman ladies were aware that it was toxic, but that didn't always stop them.

CLEO'S TIPS

Maybe women should have followed Cleopatra's example: she used the gel of aloe vera as a skin care product. She also used asses' milk to bathe in, if we are to believe the stories. Another of her beauty tricks was to dissolve crushed eggshells in vinegar for use as a calcium supplement. I wonder if she had good teeth.

Face masks were produced using lentils, honey, barley, legumes or fennel. These could be added to rose essence or myrrh. More unusual ingredients included deer horns, kingfisher droppings, mouse, placenta and other nasty bits of the body, bile, or calves' urine. These ingredients were blended into oils or goose grease, along with basil juice, oregano seeds, hawthorn, sulphur, honey and vinegar. I can see why the rose oil or myrrh was needed.

HAIR CARE

Roman men were obsessed with preventing baldness, and kept their beards well-groomed in barber shops. They used fragrances as well, especially during ceremonies. Like the Egyptians, Roman men also removed excess hair from their bodies. A slave was assigned to the baths to assist in male depilation.

Greying hair was also something to be avoided. Pliny's recorded remedy for greying hair was to shave the head, stay in the shade and then smear the head with a crow's egg, beaten in a copper vase. Dark hair could be enriched or enhanced by using black antimony mixed with animal fat, wormwood mixed in rose oil or cooked cypress leaves saturated in vinegar. Red hair was kept that way using henna and blond hair was maintained by using a potion of goat's fat and beech ash. Ladies of less virtue, belonging to the oldest profession, had brighter orange or red hair. They were called prostitutes of Rufae, which means red. Deep blue could also be achieved, probably obtained from the indigo plant. Men also dyed their hair for fashion. At one stage blonde was popular and one emperor was said to have sprinkled his hair with gold powder.

CARE FOR SOME NEW HAIR?

Wigs became elaborate, and hairstyles were enhanced with hairpieces. Imperial wigs were made using real human hair. Black and dark-coloured hair was imported from India, and blondes or lighter shades were supplied from Barbarian women's hair, from Northern Europe. Wigs made it possible for Roman women to keep up with the fashion. They also covered up the damage caused by hair dyes or hid the dreaded grey.

A Byzantine physician in the fifth and sixth century AD left a list of ancient pharmacopoeia. A toning tonic for breasts suggested the taking of plantain when the moon was in descent and applying it to the breasts. Another recipe included alum, castor oil and red wine. So far, so good. Unfortunately the addition of white lead pigment doesn't sound so wholesome.

Beauty cases were made from wood and containers were made from hand-blown glass. Amber was sometimes used to mould them together. Inside there would be an array of lipstick and eye make-up. The case also held perfume vials. These were sealed shut and had to be broken at one end, in order to be opened. Perhaps this is how the perfume described by the historian and naturalist, Pliny, in the first century AD, kept so fresh for eight years. Modern distillation of perfume was not invented until centuries later.

Women continued to highlight their brows with powders made from antimony, a metallic element. Lampblack, fine black soot created by the burning of certain materials, was used mainly as a pigment. They coloured their eyelids with green shadows obtained, like the Egyptians, from malachite or with blues from azurite, another soft copper carbonate mineral. Fuco, a red algae from the mulberry, was probably better for you than some mineral substances such as cinnabar or red mercury, red plaster and miniate (paint with red lead). Mixed with animal extracts, these were turned into red-toned lipsticks. I expect it was fine until your lips or face fell off!

Toothpastes were made by blending pumice powder with bicarbonate of soda. Bad breath was treated with pills made by the perfume makers.

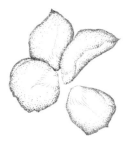

PERFUMES

Of course, the Queen of Perfume was really Cleopatra (69–30 BC). Her liaison with Marc Anthony is well documented, and she wrote about the art of make-up and cosmetics. She opened centres along the shores of the Dead Sea. Unfortunately her works were later lost and are only now known through Roman references.

En Gedi, the largest oasis along the western shore of the Dead Sea, is an area 400 metres (1,300 feet) below sea level. Salt concentrations were very high due to frequent evaporation of water. Excavations have uncovered nine separate rooms, including a waiting room furnished with stone benches. Preserved pools were used for treating plants needed in perfume- making. The centre produced what Pliny refers to as '*Asphalite*', a mud known as black tar. This was extracted from petroleum, and used to cure skin complaints. The Dead Sea salts were used as medications as well as in cosmetic recipes. This may have been the first beauty spa. In addition, persimmon plantations, confiscated for Cleopatra by Marc Anthony, provided the fruit for a perfume that is said to have driven men to madness. The resin collected was used for a famous perfume of the times. Engravings discovered on a synagogue floor in En Gedi provide a warning not to reveal the secret of the perfume's production. The modern equivalent of persimmon is not known. See a later section for more up to date Dead Sea spa treatments.

With the conquering of Egypt in 332 BC, Alexander the Great created the major trading centre for spices coming from the Orient to Europe. He had a special interest in parts of Africa where many aloes grew and is said to have used them to help heal the wounds of his soldiers. Alexandria, on the Mediterranean coast of Egypt, was a spice trading centre, where African and Asian spice traders conducted their trade with their western counterparts. Persian traders carried, among other things, cinnamon, roses, orris root and the gum resins frankincense and myrrh. Caravans came from India, China and South-East Asia. These were taken by ship across the Greek and Roman Mediterranean. Alexandria shipped to Rome and other cities, where the top manufactures of perfumes developed.

After Rome took over Egypt in 30 BC, there was an even greater flood of spices into the Mediterranean from India via the Red sea canal and then on to Greece and Italy.

Perfumes were mostly plant based. Roots, blossoms or leaves of henna, cinnamon, turpentine, iris, lilies, roses and bitter almonds, to name but a few, were soaked in oil and sometimes cooked. The essence was extracted by squeezing, just like in Egyptian times, and oil was added to produce liquid perfumes. Creams and salves were made by adding wax or fat. Many perfumes had more than a dozen ingredients. Essence of rose petals was produced in the town of Palestrina on the outskirts of Rome. Various species of lilies were used as well as myrtle, laurel, jasmine and quince. Essences became valuable commodities, with staggering price tags. Egypt supplied an expensive perfume called Judean balsam.

The Romans did not enjoy the messy processing of scented oils and imported most of theirs from Egypt. Men and women bathed in fragrance and sweethearts were often referred to as 'my myrrh, my cinnamon,' just as today 'honey' or 'love' might be used as terms of endearment.

The Greeks especially liked to use scented oils. Hippocrates recommended their use in the bath. Proprietors of *unguentarii* shops sold marjoram, lily, thyme, sage, anise, rose and iris infused in oil. Beeswax was used for thickening. Unguents were sold in elaborately decorated pots. These soothers were sold for a multitude of medicinal uses and for personal pleasure and sensuality. Men used a different scented oil for each part of their body. For example, warm and stimulating mint was used for the arms. Oils were also used to massage tight muscles. In India and later in Greece and Rome, specially prepared oils were applied before and after participating in athletic events.

EASTERN OILS AND PERFUMES

In the Indian Ayurvedic tradition women used jasmine on their hands, patchouli on the neck and cheeks and amber on their breasts. Spikenard is a member of the Valerian family and grows in the Himalayas. It is also referred to as nard, the oil of which is used for perfume, incense and herbal medicine. The Greeks also used nard, which is similar to lavender. It was treated as a luxury and in Rome it was the main ingredient of the perfume *nardinium*. Pliny's *Natural History* lists twelve species of nard. Nard is mentioned in the Bible: twice in the *Song of Solomon*. A woman anointed Jesus's head with nard and Mary, sister of Lazarus, used pure nard to anoint His feet.

Spikenard was rubbed into the hair by Indian women. Musk was used on the abdomen, sandalwood on the thighs and saffron on the feet. Men only used sandalwood. Daily bathing in India required the application of sesame oils scented with jasmine, coriander, cardamom, basil, costus, pandanus, agarwood, pine, saffron, champac and clove. Ancient

Vedic books gave instruction on the use of such aromas and some therapeutic uses have passed on to other parts of the world.

Women in India still use a cream that included turmeric, flour or wheat husk mixed with milk. The wheat husk would remove dead cell tissue, just like more modern natural body scrubs containing oatmeal. Turmeric is known toady as a very interesting and medicinally beneficial spice.

Patchouli was grown in China around 2,000 years ago. It is a base in several perfumes for both men and women. There are about eighty species in South-East Asia. It became popular in the west during the middle of the nineteenth century, when the first dried leaves arrived in London. Before that, it was a well-known fragrance in Indian textiles throughout Europe and is used as an insect repellent. See the A to Z section.

SOUTH AMERICAN OILS

Massage with scented oils was used as therapy and treatment. One massage oil prepared by the Incas contained valerian and other herbs, thickened with seaweed. The Aztecs massaged those who were ill with scented ointments.

JAPANESE GEISHA MAKE-UP

The make-up of traditional geisha, or female entertainers and performers, once contained rice powder, lead and mercury. This could turn a geisha 's skin yellow and give her lead poisoning. The white powder foundation, oshiroi, later included zinc, glycerine and titanium oxide. Young geishas wear heavier make-up whereas more experienced and older women wear less. The white make-up is less frequently used today than in the past. The process started with sticks of waxy oils being applied to the face, similar to that used by sumo wrestlers in their hair, followed by the white powder mixed with water to form a paste. A few areas of the face and neck are left unpainted to give the look of a mask instead of natural skin. The make-up covers the face, neck and chest with two or three V- or W-shaped areas left on the nape of the neck.

Lipstick made of crushed safflower petals was used to paint the eyebrows and eyes as well as the lips. Crystallised sugar helped to add lustre to the lips and the actual application of the lip colour and extent helped to define status. The lower lip is coloured in partially and the upper lip left white for some geisha, and newly trained geisha will only colour the top lip fully. Charcoal was also used. Rouge contoured the eye sockets and black paint coloured the teeth for the ceremony marking the end of a geisha's training.

CHINESE FRAGRANCE

Chinese people are said to have stained their fingernails with gum arabic, wax and egg for thousands of years. The colours used represented social class, ranging from gold, silver, black and white for the upper classes and muted colours for the lower classes, who were forbidden to use bright colours.

As the soldiers of the Crusades of the Middle Ages returned from the East with oils and spices, fragrances such as rose-water and solid perfumes travelled across Europe. Trade with China saw a huge increase in the use of herbs and spices. From the seventh century China had been using scent quite freely. As well as baths, clothes, buildings, paper and ink were perfumed. Taoists believed that extraction of a plant's fragrance liberated its soul. Like the Greeks, the Chinese used one word, *heang*, to represent perfume, incense and fragrance. Six aesthetic moods were identified, broadly described as tranquil, reclusive, luxurious, beautiful, refined or noble.

Between the seventh and seventeenth centuries the Chinese upper classes were mad on fragrance, using scented wood to make statues and fans. Sachets of fragrance would be thrown at audiences during dance performances. Along with jasmine oils from India, Persian rose-water, Indonesian cloves, ginger, nutmeg and patchouli were used extensively. In the thirteenth century, when Marco Polo established trade between China and Italy, he opened up a lucrative trade between the two countries.

The great wealth of Venice at the time is said to have originated from the spice trade. Spices were transported to the north on overland routes by pack horse up the Rhone Valley and later, after the early thirteenth century, by galley to the ports of Holland, Germany, France, Belgium and England. The later explorations of Columbus, financed by Spain, and the Portuguese voyages of discovery, which eventually established a route to India, finally opened up the world spice trade.

DYING TO LOOK YOUR BEST

In the western world cosmetics didn't really become known until the Middle Ages and were only then available for the rich. The absence of regulation over the following centuries to the manufacture and use of cosmetics led to deformities, blindness and death. White lead, used to cover the face during the Renaissance, was one example.

The damage inflicted by the lead was unintentional, but arsenic in face powder was a different story.

DEAD GOOD, THIS WATER

Aqua Toffana, named after its creator Signora Toffana, was a poison sold as a cosmetic and designed for women from rich families. During the mid-seventeenth century Toffana and her daughter made a good living from the product. She was sympathetic to the low status of women and often sold her potion to women trapped in difficult marriages. She received many referrals, some totally innocent but many of her customers purchased it with intent to poison. The victim could then die 'accidentally'. *Aqua Toffana* contained mostly arsenic and lead and possibly belladonna. It was a colourless, tasteless liquid that could easily be mixed with water or wine to be served during meals. The container directed women to visit the inventor for proper instructions. During the visit, women would be told never to drink the make-up, but to apply it to their cheeks when their husbands were around. Over 600 victims are known to have died from this poison: most were the husbands of unhappy spouses.

PALE-FACE BEAUTIES

European women in the Middle Ages followed the pale-face trend set by the Greeks and Romans. Women who had to work outdoors acquired a suntan and those who didn't wanted to show off their affluence by being pale. Some fashionable sixth-century women are said to have achieved the look by bleeding themselves.

As a contrast, Spanish prostitutes wore pink make-up to set themselves apart from the pallor of high-class women's faces. Thirteenth-century Italian women wore pink lipstick to show that they were wealthy enough to afford synthetic make-up. Was nobody ever satisfied? No change there, then!

ELIZABETHAN COSMETICS

SLAP IT ON WITH A TROWEL

The idea of beauty in Elizabethan times is well represented by portraits of Queen Elizabeth and her contemporaries. In the sixteenth century standards of beauty called for a small, rosy mouth along with a straight, narrow nose and wide-set, bright eyes. Women would use poisonous belladonna in their eyes to achieve a bright sparkle. Powdered antimony or kohl enhanced the size of the eyes. Plucked eyebrows were a must for court ladies, as was a high brow, which was supposed to be a sign of aristocracy. Women would pluck their hairline back an inch or more to create a high forehead.

Pale skin with an alabaster complexion was achieved at great cost. In a time when skin problems were commonplace and sunscreen was unknown, smooth, unblemished and pale skin was extremely rare. Ceruse, a mixture of white lead and vinegar, created a white foundation that was applied to the face, neck and chest. First recorded in the 1520s, it was well established by the time Elizabeth became queen. One recipe involved mixing lead with ground marble and heating it in a kiln for several days. The residue was ground up and mixed with figs and vinegar to make a thick paste. This concoction would slowly burn away the surface of the skin.

Many warned of the skin problems this would cause and suggested alternatives made from, among other substances, alum and tin ash, sulphur, boiled egg white and talc.

Beeswax, asses' milk and powdered jawbones of hogs also featured. Nice!

Egg white was also used to give a glazed finish and help hide wrinkles. Sometimes false veins were traced on to the thickly applied make-up to accentuate the pallor.

Blusher and lip colouring were made by grinding down a bright red mineral called cinnabar. Madder root, cochineal and ochre-based compounds were all used to tint for rouge and lip colour. Vermilion, or mercuric sulphide, which is deadly if swallowed, was the popular choice of the fashionable court lady. One satirist of the day commented that an artist did not need a box of paints to work from, but merely a fashionably painted lady standing nearby to use for pigments.

Such heavy and often poisonous make-up caused serious skin damage. Remedies ranged from the application of lemon juice or rose-water to even more worrying concoctions including mercury, alum, honey and eggshells. Washing the face with mercury was a common facial peel. Look, no face left!

Blonde or reddish hair was eagerly sought after. Decidedly dodgy recipes for bleaching hair existed, including the use of urine. If the colour wasn't right, or the hair had been damaged beyond repair, a woman could always wear a wig. This was a lot easier than struggling with their own hair. Women strove hard to copy the Queen's look of tightly curled red hair at the front and pale colouring.

PUMICE TOOTHPASTE

Elizabeth's teeth were badly decayed by the time of her death. She may well have used a popular toothpaste made from ground pumice stone, which got rid of plaque, but also removed the enamel, exposing them to even more rapid decay. Honeyed and sweetened foods probably didn't help either.

MUSK

Washing or bathing were not high on the agenda for the Queen and court, so strong scents and perfume were essential. Spicy scents such as nutmeg and rosemary were in vogue and one popular perfume of the time was made from rose-water, ambergris and civet musk. Interestingly, or worryingly, civet is still highly valued as a fragrance and stabilising agent for perfume today. It can be harvested by either killing the animal and removing the anal glands, or by scraping the secretions from the live animal. At least one major perfume manufacturer claims to have used a synthetic substitute since 1998. What took so long?

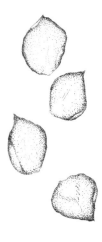

18TH- AND 19TH-CENTURY COSMETICS

By the seventeenth century Europe was still recovering from bouts of illness such as smallpox, which left survivors with nasty, pockmarked scars. Deep pits were left by pustules drying out. This is perhaps why thick white make-up prevailed, in order to hide the scars. During the eighteenth century things changed dramatically. The use of rouge became a class indicator. Only bad girls used it. Prostitutes put it on their lips and cheeks to mimic the effects of sexual arousal. They also wore it on their nipples and other areas.

In France during the eighteenth century, rouge and lipstick were all the rage and suggested a healthy and lively spirit. People in other countries, however, became tired of excessive make-up and even suggested that the French must be unattractive and have something to hide. Rouge (the French word for 'red') was created from unwholesome ingredients, including carmine, a lead-based pigment, and plaster of Paris. Fashionable red spots on the cheeks made a contrast to a pale, powdered face. Rouge was available as a lipstick for men and women.

18TH-CENTURY HAIRSTYLES

These subjected men's and women's hair to various tortures. One of the least harmful was probably powdering the hair after curling it with hot tongs. A base of lard was applied for the powder to stick to. Big hair and complicated styling was the order of the day, to complement fashionable clothing. Many people wore hairpieces and wigs to add volume to their hair. These were difficult to attach and maintain on a daily basis, so women often had their hair done once every few weeks and left it unwashed so that it would stay that way. Women suffered, unsurprisingly, from scalp problems and infestations of lice and fleas. It is said that some fashion victims found mice nesting in their hair because the pork fat had attracted them. Stylish!

POMADE

Hair pomades were made from cleaned pork fat and wax, scented with essential oils. The more beeswax they contained, the greater the stiffness could be achieved. They gave a shiny, slick appearance unless powdered. Unlike modern hair spray and gels, pomade doesn't dry and takes several washes to remove. Some pomades are still made today and I was interested to learn that special shampoo can be used, as well as olive oil and cola. Petroleum jelly is a main constituent, or can be used on its own. Mineral oil and wax are also used, along with perfume and colouring agents. The stiffest will have a higher proportion of beeswax.

FRAGRANCE AND CLEANSING

The Crusaders brought alcohol-based perfumes to Europe. The first modern perfume was created in 1370, at the command of Queen Elizabeth of Hungary. It was made of scented oils blended in an alcohol solution and was known as Hungary water. France quickly cottoned on and became a centre for perfume, cultivating vast amounts of flowers for their essence. By the eighteenth century, aromatic plants were being grown especially for the purpose in the Grasse region of France. These provided the growing perfume industry with raw materials.

Scented waters, sometimes made with leftovers from distilling essential oils such as cinnamon and cloves, were used for washing and for perfuming other cosmetics. Various citrus fruit spirits were added to an assortment of Mediterranean herbs, roses and violets and spices such as cardamom to scent the pomades.

Vinegars scented with elder, amber and musk were probably used for skin cleansing and to compensate for the soap used in occasional washing of the hair. Various skincare and cleansing substances such as cleansing milk, lotions and creams were available. Tooth powders and tinctures were around, as were colourings for hair and wigs.

POWDERS AND PATCHES

Powders were popular, probably because creams tended to go bad without preservatives or refrigeration. To avoid spillage, white paints were mixed with a bonding agent and rolled into balls for drying. When required, the balls could be ground back to powder and applied to the face or hair. The metal oxides used to achieve the white powder were mostly harmful. Talc was not so effective at covering up, so lead, bismuth, pewter and mercury were all used.

Another way to cover up the odd large pit or pockmark was to wear a small patch made from fabric, which was stuck on to the face and upper chest, like beauty spots.

They could be shaped as stars, moons, hearts or anything of your choice. A type of communication developed from their use. A patch near the mouth meant you were flirtatious and you could also signal whether you were married, available or otherwise by their position elsewhere on the face. Hopefully, they would still cover the scars up as well!

CLASSICAL LOOK

By the end of the century, following the French Revolution, more realistic fashion changes took hold in Europe. The female fashion was to wear a wig of curling coils on top while allowing the natural hair to fall loosely down the neck.

Roman and Greek fashions returned, with cropped simple hairstyles for men. The simplicity of freshly washed hair noted on Greek artefacts was thought to be more attractive.

CHANGES IN SOAP MANUFACTURE

As we know, soap is basically a reaction between fatty acids and an alkaki (lye). When fats or oils are mixed with a strong alkali, the fats are split into fatty acids and glycerine. About 7–13 per cent of a mix will be glycerine. Up until the late nineteenth century people didn't know how to recover glycerine from the soap-making process. Most commercially produced glycerine came from the candle-making industry, where candles were still made from animal fats. Glycerine was mostly used to make nitro glycerine and dynamite. Interestingly, soap manufacture became a much more lucrative business to invest in at about this time. Could there be a connection, I wonder?

Early soap manufacturers obtained the lye from putting potash into a bottomless barrel over a stone slab, resting on rocks. Straw or sticks were put in the bottom as a sort of sieve. By slowly pouring water over the ashes you could produce the lye, a brown liquid dripping down into a container below. This could then be used with the rendered down fat to produce soap. When wood supplies dwindled towards the end of the eighteenth century, pearlash manufacturing started to decline, making way for more commercial methods. The Leblanc process, invented in the late eighteenth century, changed soap making for ever. Sodium alkalis made harder, better soap without the necessity to add salt.

SOAP AND GLYCERINE MANUFACTURE

Fats and oils are heated with caustic soda to produce soap and glycerine. The continuous process, developed in about 1940, means as the name suggests, that production can continue without making batches. Soap takes about six hours to make nowadays. Previously, by the 'kettle process', it took four to eleven days to complete a batch.

Soap and glycerine are produced as the fat reacts with alkali after boiling. To separate the soap and glycerine, salt is added, causing the soap to rise to the top and the glycerine to settle to the bottom.

VICTORIAN ATTITUDES TO COSMETICS

In the nineteenth century a natural look became fashionable. Excessive make-up denoted the mark of a loose woman. Most men believed women wore no make-up, but cosmetic were available and beauty books gave advice. Lip and cheek rouge were considered too much and women were encouraged to bite their lips and pinch their cheeks before entering a room. Commercial make-up from France included powders, bases and waxes containing light, natural colour. Cold cream was sold for removal of make-up and anti-ageing creams and wrinkle cures were advertised. One suggestion for the latter was that women should sleep with their face bound in strips of raw beef. Tasty!

Women in nineteenth-century society were supposed to be fragile and delicate. 'Pale and interesting' marked gentility and social status. This could be achieved by drinking vinegar and avoiding fresh air. Parasols were used to protect faces outside and heavy curtains kept the sun out of the house. Low necklines were for evening exposure only. Obvious make-up was frowned upon and only discreet use was made of a little rouge on the cheeks. As Queen Victoria's reign progressed, social etiquette became more rigid. Actresses such as Sarah Bernhardt and Lillie Langtry used make-up, but the Queen was not amused or tempted herself. Most cosmetic products were still either of dubious chemical origin or were concocted in the kitchen with food colourings, berries and beetroot dye. Hair was natural, long and rarely cut. False hairpieces were used on occasion.

MOTHER HUBBARD

In the 1880s, Harriet Hubbard Ayer promoted face creams and beauty advice through her work in New York. She marketed a cream under the name of Madame Recamier, a famous beauty from French Napoleonic times. She seems to have been a colourful character and shrewd businesswoman, despite family problems when her daughter and her ex-husband had her committed to a mental asylum. This only stopped her for a year, however. Her advice wasn't all bad either. She explained the need for hair care and the reasons why hair might fall out. She was also sensitive to the problems of facial hair in women, although couldn't provide much help. Her suggestions that diet caused spots may have been unusual at the time, but she recommended avoiding tea, coffee, cocoa, chocolate, sweets, pork and buckwheat cakes in favour of fruits, green vegetables, celery, watercress, spinach and hot water.

Sulphur soap was recommended, as were saline purgatives, ointment of tar, lanolin and sulphur baths. She estimated that, at the turn of the century, twenty million dollars per year were spent on cosmetics and cures in the USA and suggested that, although American women were not stupid, they were at least gullible. All they needed to do was stop eating pie and cakes! Some things never change.

Perfume also came under the scrutiny of Mrs Hubbard Ayer, who marketed her own. She bemoaned the fact that oils and pomades had not improved and that Eastern perfumes made hundreds of years ago could not be bettered. She gave instruction as to how to express essential oils from flowers and plants, and suggested violet, honeysuckle, tuberose, jonquil, jasmine, narcissus, orange flowers and myrtle blossoms as the best American plants to use instead of trapping their smell in fat.

She recommended buying costly essential oil or pomade from a reputable supplier. One ounce (25 g) of pomade could make 16 oz (450 g) of extract. All you needed was a pint of pure alcohol, mixed with the oil in a clean bottle. This was to be heated to 85°F (29.5°C) in hot water before closing the bottle securely. Like good wine, this apparently improved with keeping and a few drops would knock your socks off.

The twentieth century brought about safety standards in the use of cosmetics, but with much wider scope for ingredients, both natural and synthetic. It is also where a new set of problems began for those sensitive to some of these synthetic additives. It became popular to have tanned, healthy looking skin. That, of course, opens up a whole new discussion on the rights and wrongs of excessive exposure to the sun, but this is where the history of natural cosmetics ends for the time being.

AN A TO Z
OF
NATURAL
INGREDIENTS

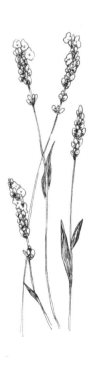

AN A TO Z OF NATURAL INGREDIENTS

This section offers a brief summary of many ingredients, animal, mineral and vegetable, that can be used as natural cosmetics. It is by no means exhaustive and inclusion on the list is not meant to be read as a recommendation. If there is any doubt as to whether a plant or ingredient might be right for a specific remedy or treatment, expert advice should be taken. Some of the ingredients, such as petroleum jelly and glycerine, are not strictly 'natural', as they have been produced by industrial methods. They are included because of their widespread use in the making of natural cosmetics. Knowing what a product is made from might help you choose when trying to avoid certain ingredients. Some sections are fuller than others, reflecting personal knowledge and experience.

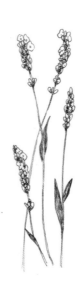

Acacia, Arabic Gum, Gum Tree (*Acacia arabica, Acacia nilotica*)

This is a tree with fragrant, golden-yellow flowers. Long, white seed pods contain saponin. The bark yields several polyphenolic compounds, including, quercetin, sucrose and tannin. Quercetin is part of the pigment also found in the skins of apples and red onions and is a powerful antioxidant, natural anti-histamine and anti-inflammatory. Gum made from pieces of the plant dissolved in water is a demulcent and protects inflamed surfaces.

(*Acacia concina, Acacia sinuata*)

These varieties are sometimes referred to as soap plants because they contain saponin. However, many other species of plants around the world are also called soap plants. See soapberry, below.

Saponins dissolve in water to create a soapy froth (sapon actually means 'soap'); they are mild detergents used commercially and are also useful for astringent and cleansing action. Saponin is not for internal consumption and can be poisonous. It is said to be very good for external use, promoting hair growth and having an anti-dundruff effect. But, as always, if in doubt, don't use it.

Acacia farnesiana is used in the perfume industry due to its strong fragrance. Acacia has been used as a fragrance for centuries. Biblical references include the burning of acacia wood as a form of incense.

Aloe Vera (*Aloe Vera* L. *Burm*)

Various parts of this useful perennial plant are used. Leaf, juice, gel and dried powder products are available from suppliers. There are at least 275 species of aloe (some claim up to 400) that belong to the lily family, although only aloe vera is used for cosmetics. Aloes are closely related to garlic, onions and asparagus. The short stem and shallow root system support fleshy leaves in rosettes. The leaves retain water in dry hot climates, as this plant is a succulent. When a leaf is cut a yellow, bitter sap escapes. This sap was used as a laxative in the past, although I wouldn't recommend trying it. I'm not sure I'd want to use home grown aloe either, as this yellow sap gets in the way of the gel, which is the really good part. The gel is found under the skin of the leaves. The sap acts as a deterrent to insects and predators and may contaminate a recipe, leading to complications.

Aloe vera has great moisturising properties and is excellent for the skin. It is also claimed as an anti-ageing formula. The pH value is very close to that of skin. A complex group of biologically active chemicals and enzymes account for its properties. The gel is used in a number of ways for skin care. Anti-inflammatory properties alleviate the pain and swelling associated with itches and burns. Aloe vera has proved beneficial in the treatment of eczema, psoriasis, dermatitis, abrasions to the skin, acne and sunburn. Its moisturising properties are well documented and the gel contains amino acids, minerals, vitamins and proteins. Some people claim relief from applying gel to minor burns. The gel consists of less than 1 per cent solids containing polysaccharides. The rest is all water and the water retaining capacity of the gel helps to cool the skin.

Almond (*Prunus dulcis*)
This is the sweet almond, high in fatty acids, and an excellent emollient that helps to soften and soothe the skin while preventing moisture loss. Bitter almond

oil cannot be used for cosmetics, as it contains traces of a form of cyanide. Sweet almond oil is easily absorbed into the skin without leaving a greasy feel. It is used to soften the skin and to promote a clear, youthful complexion. It is obtained from the dried kernels of the almond tree.

Amla (*Indian Gooseberry*)
Amla is said to contain 20 times more vitamin C than orange juice. It nourishes and thickens the hair, apparently by penetrating the scalp and strengthening the roots. It is an excellent conditioning herb. Amla oil has been used in Indian medicine for centuries to treat scalp problems. It is used in shampoos and conditioning rinses as well as in hair pomades and oil treatments. See also *Eclipta alba,* below.

Apricot
Fresh or dried apricot fruit moisturises dry skin and provides vitamin A. The crushed kernels can be used with a loofah to exfoliate the skin. These should only be used externally. My biggest problem with apricots, however, is that even the smell of them makes me nauseous, so they're not on my personal list of favourites. Mashed, fresh or dried apricots can be mixed with warm olive oil to form a paste.

Apricot kernel oil is a popular massage oil and carrier oil when combined with essential oils for aromatherapy. It contains vitamin A and can relieve itching and dry skin. Apricot oil is said to be good for lip balm.

Arrowroot
Arrowroot is used in talcum powders and hair dyes. It is added to moisturisers as a thickening agent, although it doesn't appear to have any beneficial or harmful effects on the skin. Similar to cornflour,

it makes a very fine white powder. I don't ever remember coming across arrowroot apart from as an easily digestible food or my mum using it as a topping for fruit flans when I was a child. It can apparently be mixed with cornflour as a safer alternative to talc, which is synthetic (see below). It can be used to help dry up blemishes and rashes. American Indians used it to heal wounds, such as those caused by poisoned arrows. It can be mixed with dried camomile as a prickly heat treatment.

Avocado (*Persea Americana*)
This fruit, a native of Mexico, Central and Southern America, is now widely grown in tropical and subtropical climates, and is a rich source of vitamins A, D and E. Avocado oil stabilises emulsions and is a good carrier oil. It is used in cleansing creams, soaps, shampoos, moisturisers, lipstick, bath oils and sunscreen products. It has antibacterial properties and can treat minor skin irritation. Like cocoa butter and almond oil, it is high in fatty acids and is especially recommended for mature skin.

Basil (*Ocimum basilicum*)
Basil is an easily grown herb that is widely used in food as well as cosmetics, perfumes, shampoos and soaps. It is used to restore lustre to dull, limp hair. Basil is also claimed to have anti-ageing properties containing ursolic acid, which improves the health of skin and hair. It is claimed to improve the appearance of wrinkles and age spots by restoring the skin's collagen and elasticity. Maybe I should try it. I eat enough of it!

Beeswax
Beeswax contains compounds which are also found in human skin and is a hydrating compound that helps to

increase moisture. An ingredient of many hand and body creams, it is also used as a conditioner and UV inhibitor. It appears in lip gloss, most lipsticks and a range of face creams and ointments. The wax is produced by young bees from twelve to eighteen days old. They cluster together in large numbers to increase their body temperature. After having consumed large amounts of honey they slowly excrete slivers of wax about the size of a pinhead. Other bees then harvest the wax for use in sealing cells. To produce a pound of wax, bees eat 2.7 kilos (6 lb) of honey. The wax is filtered and cleaned for cosmetic use and the colour reflects the flowers and nectar the honey was made from. See also, Honey and Royal Jelly.

Bergamot (*Citrus aurantium bergamia*)
This is a small and roughly pear-shaped citrus fruit, grown mainly in Italy. The trees are a cross between a pear lemon and a Seville orange or a grapefruit. The peel of the fruit is used extensively in the perfume industry because the scented oil combines well with other fragrances. About a third of all perfumes contain bergamot oil, which has obvious lemony tones. The original eau de Cologne was created in the seventeenth century using bergamot. I never get tired of this smell. Bergamot oil can be used for a range of skin problems and irritations.

Bicarbonate of Soda
One of the many beneficial uses of this natural mineral relate to cleansing and odour reduction.
Did you know that the main ingredient in fizzy bath products is bicarbonate of soda? You can make your own with three parts bicarbonate of soda to one part citric acid. Add your own fragrance oils or colouring (see recipe section). Here are some uses:

○ After brushing with toothpaste, apply a little bicarbonate of soda to the toothbrush and re-brush your teeth. This will help to whiten them.
○ Dust the armpits with bicarbonate of soda after washing or showering.
○ Apply a paste of bicarbonate of soda with a drop of water to spots and leave for about ten minutes. Rinse off carefully with warm water but never rub or scrub your skin.
○ Soak tired, smelly feet in a bowl of hot water with four tablespoons of bicarbonate of soda. The soaking will soften hard skin, which you can remove with a pumice stone.
○ After painting, gutting fish or preparing onions, get rid of the lingering odour with a sprinkling of bicarbonate of soda on your hands. Rub them together before washing with soapy water.
○ Wash hairbrushes and combs in a solution of bicarbonate of soda and warm water to remove build-up of products.
○ Use one part bicarbonate of soda to one part sea salt in a hot bath. Lie back and relax for 20 minutes. Rinse off or shower to remove the salt.
○ As a water softener use half a cup of bicarbonate of soda in the bath, and add to running water.

Calendula (marigold)
Calendula petals can be used to make a skin cream or cleanser. A strong infusion made from marigold petals can be used to lighten fair hair. The flowers are used for hair rinse and herbal baths. Calendula can be mixed with camomile and comfrey for a soothing application for all skin types. As a bonus, marigold perfume keeps flies away! During the American Civil War it was used to treat wounds. It can be used both internally and externally.

Camphor (*Cinnamomum camphora*)
Camphor oil is a preservative commonly found in cosmetics, haircare products, emollients and astringents. It leaves the skin feeling cool and fresh. In India the oil is used to treat acne and inflammation.

Carob (*Ceratonia siliqua*)
Carob gum is used in food products as well as moisturisers, anti-ageing creams, foundation and around-eye creams. Carob seed-pod flour is used in the manufacture of herbal facepacks, which have a cleansing and toning effect on the skin. It is also used in face powder, as a breath freshener and nail treatment.

Carnauba (*Copernicia prunifera*)
This comes from the leaves of the carnauba palm in Brazil. It is usually sold as hard yellowy flakes. It is used in a number of glossy wax finishes, including car waxes, furniture polish (when mixed with beeswax) and dental floss. In cosmetics it appears in lipsticks, eyeliners and mascara, eye shadows, foundations and skincare preparations, amongst other things.

Centella (*Indian pennywort, gotu kala*)
This small trailing herb, *Centella asiatica,* has been used traditionally in the management of skin disorders. The extract has been included in anti-ageing creams and other topical formulations for sensitive and dry skin as well as in the treatment of stretch marks. When added to a facial mask it is said to rejuvenate and regenerate the skin and strengthen the tissues.

Chamomile/Babuna (*Maticia chamomile*)
Chamomile is one of the most popular herbal

remedies in the world and is used in a variety of applications. Its volatile oils are used in cosmetic creams and lotions and it is often combined with other herbs such as lavender to create aromatic bath-time treats. Chamomile tones, calms and soothes the skin. It has antibacterial properties and also contains anti-histamine and digestive properties. Chamomile appears in skin lotions, shampoo for blondes, cleansers and other products. An infusion of chamomile is used to treat irritated and inflamed skin and also to rinse blonde hair, as it acts as a lightener. Some people swear by camomile tea as a soothing drink.

Cinnamon (*Cinnamomum zeylanicum*)
Despite being widely used in food, aromatherapy and pharmacy, cinnamon is also important in the perfume industries. Although cinnamon bark is mildly astringent, it has few cosmetic uses, being strongly stimulating to the skin. It is toning and warming.

Citrus oils
Because of their concentrated nature, essential oils generally should not be applied directly to the skin in an undiluted form. They should be blended with a vegetable carrier oil such as olive, almond or grape seed oil. Many citrus oils increase the skin's reaction to sunlight and make it more likely to burn. See also bergamot and lemons.

Cocoa butter
Cocoa butter comes from the roasted seeds of the cocoa plant. It is one of the most stable fats and contains antioxidants that allow for a long storage life. It is full of fatty acids that include about a quarter palmitic acid, about a third stearic acids and a similar amount of oleic acid. Palmitic acid is a major component of the oil from palm trees. Stearic

acid is a waxy solid, used in confectionery and also in making candles, soaps, plastics, oil pastels and cosmetics, and for softening rubber. (See below). Oleic acid is a monounsaturated omega-9 fatty acid. Cocoa butter is water repellent and helpful for dry skin. It also has some sunblocking properties.

Cocoa powder
Cocoa powder is full of antioxidants and helps to soften oily skin. Natural cocoa is light in colour and somewhat acidic, with a pH of 5.2–5.8. Cocoa is the dried and partially fermented fatty seed of the cacao tree from which chocolate is made. Cocoa powder is made by grinding cocoa seeds and removing the cocoa butter from the dark, bitter cocoa solids.

Cornflour
Made from finely ground maize, this everyday kitchen ingredient can be used as a substitute for talcum powder. Cornflour absorbs moisture and oil residues, giving a matte finish. It can be used for nappy rash or underarm, neck or other areas where moisture accumulates. With the addition of a few drops of essential oil it provides a luxurious dusting powder.

Cucumber (*Cucumis sativus*)
Cucumber is good for rubbing over the skin to keep it soft. Cucumber juice is cooling, healing and soothing to the skin and improves moisture retention. A cucumber wash applied to the skin after exposure to winds is said to be extremely beneficial.

Eclipta alba (*false daisy or Bhringraj*)
A black dye obtained from *Eclipta alba* is used for dyeing hair and tattooing. This plant also has other, traditional external uses such as for treating athlete foot, eczema and dermatitis. In ayurvedic medicine,

the leaf extract is considered especially good for the hair and it is applied to the scalp to address hair loss. A preparation made with amla and *eclipta alba* is well known in India as Amla Bhringraj oil, which is used to darken the hair.

Egg
Egg yolk is a good emollient and water-binding agent for skin. Egg white, or albumen, was widely used in historical times. Eggs are often added to facials. I prefer to eat mine, in moderation!

Mix an egg yolk with a teaspoon of vinegar, a teaspoon of lemon juice and a tablespoon of olive oil. Add a teaspoon of bicarbonate of soda. Apply to the skin with circular movements. Rinse off with warm water.

Elder (*Sambucus nigra*)
This common shrub provides elderflowers that are beneficial as a skin cleanser. Elderflowers are used to make an infusion that will lighten the skin, fade freckles, soothe sunburn and make a good face pack for wrinkled skin. Elderflower eye poultices are said to be soothing as well. Alternatively you could leave the flowers to develop into berries and make wine or jam.

Evening primrose (*Oenothera*)
Evening primrose oil contains a whole range of fatty acids and anti-inflammatory properties. It was used by native North Americans to make an infusion for healing wounds. It is used in skincare for its good moisturising and emollient properties on dry skin, eczema and psoriasis.

Fennel (*Foeniculum vulgare, F. officinale*)
The properties of fennel essential oil in skincare include that of being antiseptic, soothing, cleansing and with a toning effect on mature skin. There are claims that it keeps wrinkles at bay. It reduces water retention in the skin, which can give a puffy appearance. Fennel has a spicy smell, much like aniseed, and was popular in Roman times. In high concentrations, fennel oil is not recommended for people suffering from epilepsy or for pregnant women. Ground seeds are sometimes used in face packs.

Frankincense (*Olibanum*)
Frankincense oil is extracted from resin or gum from the olibanum tree. It has antiseptic, disinfectant and astringent qualities. Frankincense has been a popular ingredient of cosmetics and incense burners since ancient Egyptian times. The Greek physician Dioscorides wrote of its properties in treating skin disorders in the first century AD. Frankincense improves skin tone and condition and the astringent qualities act as balancer of the skin, reducing dry or oily skin condition to normal. Frankincense has a woody, spicy smell, similar to camphor. It is said to strengthen gums and hair roots as well as helping to regenerate cells. It makes scars and marks left by boils or acne on the skin fade away. This apparently includes fading of stretch marks and surgery scars associated with pregnancy and delivery.

Fuller's earth
Also known as calcium bentonite, this mineral is used for acne problems and oily skin. It is sedimentary clay composed of varying amounts of aluminium, silica, iron oxides, lime, magnesia and water, in extremely variable proportions. It removes oils and impurities from the skin and produces a lightening, bleaching

effect on the outer epidermal layer. It is a useful base ingredient for facial clay recipes. I have vague recollections of using it with a mild bleach to lighten leg hair as a teenager, before I started to shave them. The effect wasn't brilliant, probably because of the lack of bleach and the fact that the skin was lightened as well the leg hair. It is probably better as a face pack ingredient. The high mineral content rejuvenates the skin while the clay exfoliates and stimulates blood circulation to the skin. Naturally occurring, coloured cosmetic clay is used in soap, lotions, creams and bath salts. Fuller's earth can be blended with jojoba oil, macadamia nut oil and rose-water, to create a facial or body mask.

Ginger (*Zingiber officinale*)
Root and dried ginger contain a wealth of beneficial compounds. Most of the benefits are derived from consuming the ginger, which also tastes great, but there are some topical uses as well. Ginger contains aromatic compounds called gingerols. Shogaols, a form of gingerols, are created as ginger ages, so the highest concentrations occur in dried ginger. Ginger is used in a huge number of traditional Chinese medicines.

Ginger oil is extracted commercially by steam distillation of dried powdered ginger, although the best ginger oil is obtained from whole, unpeeled root ginger.

Ginger oil is an oleoresin: a preparation extracted from plants that keeps the resins in solution.
The volatile oil components in ginger consist predominantly of zingeberene with curcumene and farnesene. When included in soaps, ground ginger warms the skin. It is a stimulant and anti-irritant. Its warming, soothing properties are beneficial to the skin and so ginger is an excellent ingredient for bath

oils and other cosmetics. Ginger oil is used as a fragrance in cosmetics. Here are some other uses:

- It can be diluted with massage oil and applied to skin for warming effect. Add 5–10 drops ginger oil to 25 ml (1 fl oz) almond oil for rheumatism or lumbago.
- Rashes caused by food allergies have been treated with ginger in a bath. Boil 225 g (8 oz) of fresh ginger in water and add to a bath. Have a good soak and then rinse with camomile tea.
- Athlete's foot: ginger contains antifungal compounds, so it can be administered to affected areas in a concoction twice a day. Add about 25 g (1 oz) to a cup of boiling water and let it steep for 20 minutes before applying with cotton wool.
- Chewing ginger is said to be a good mouth and breath freshener. The antibiotic properties probably see to that, and may cover up other odours, like garlic.
- The antibacterial qualities of ginger tea have been suggested for deodorising the armpits on a cloth. A shower sounds like a better idea, but in an emergency . . .
- Applied three times a week, ginger oil, lemon juice and sesame oil have been recommended for scalp complaints. Mix 1 or 2 tablespoons of ginger juice with 3 tablespoons of sesame oil and $1/2$ teaspoon lemon juice, presumably before washing the hair.
- Ginger is used in many herbal remedies to make a hot compress, but make sure it is fresh ginger.

Ginkgo (*Ginkgo biloba*)
Ginkgo is a true survivor. Four trees growing between 1–2 km ($1/2$–$1 1/4$ miles) away from the atomic bomb

exploded in Hiroshima in 1945 are still alive, whereas most life forms perished. It is known for its great revitalising, detoxifying and anti-ageing properties that give a younger looking skin. It is added to some skincare products.

Glycerine
This natural humectant can be derived from animal or vegetable fats and is used in products such as cleansers, moisturisers and soaps. It helps skin to absorb moisture by binding its structure with water, to penetrate the skin. Glycerine is a natural by-product of soap making (see the history section). It can be dissolved in water or alcohol, but not in oils, and has good emollient properties. It is one of the most popular cosmetic additives. Vegetable glycerine is usually the by-product of palm or coconut oil production, where the raw ingredients are split into crude glycerol fats. Some people are intolerant of glycerine, so its widespread use may be bad news to sufferers.

Grape seed oil (*Vitis vinifera*)
Grape seed oil is used for hair products, especially for damaged hair, and in delicate skin areas such as around the eyes, the lips and hands. It is rich in linoleic acid, which is important for skin and cell membranes. Grape seed oil acts as an emollient and moisturiser. A non-greasy oil, it acts as a good carrier for richer almond or wheat germ and is a commonly used massage oil.

Groundnut oil
See peanut oil, below.

Hemp seed oil (*Cannabis sativa*)
This has good moisturising and hydrating properties, thereby boosting lowered levels of ceramides in mature

skin. Hemp seed oil is anti-inflammatory, moisturises dry skin, helps heal skin lesions and contains anti-oxidants. The oil is non-greasy and readily absorbed. It has been used in traditional Chinese medicine for centuries.

Hemp seed oil is considered to be the most nutritional of oils, providing protein, a plethora of vitamins and minerals and fatty acids, including omega 6 and omega 3. These are important for providing lustre to skin, hair and eyes, among other things. The green colour reflects the high level of chlorophyll that is naturally present in the seeds.

Henna (*Lawsonia inermis*)
Henna is native to tropical and subtropical regions of Africa, southern Asia and northern Australasia. It has been used in India and some North African countries for centuries, but was used 5,000 years ago by the ancient Egyptians. It is used as a hair dye or in the art of Hindu mehndi patterns, in which complex designs are painted on to the hands and feet. Henna produces a red-orange dye molecule called lawsone, which bonds with protein, so it dyes skin, hair and fingernails as well as leather, silk and wool. The dye is mainly concentrated in the leaves and contains arachidic, stearic, palmitic and oleic acids. This plant extract is, therefore, a good conditioner and tonic for the hair, mostly used as a hair dye when mixed with other natural dyes. Products sold as 'black henna' are not made from henna, but may be derived from indigo. See the recipe section for hair dye information.

As a semi-permanent skin dye, henna is dried and crushed into a fine powder that is then mixed with oils and applied to the skin. The paste dries and flakes off, leaving a stain of the design of your choice in your skin that lasts for a week or longer.

Hibiscus

Hibiscus petals were used in ayurvedic medicine to stimulate thicker hair growth and to prevent premature greying and scalp disorders. Hibiscus acts as a natural hair conditioner and can be used in washes, treatments and vinegar rinses for the hair, combined with amla extract. It has also been used as a mild shampoo for babies in several parts of Polynesia and Central America. Hibiscus extract is said to promote even tone to skin affected by cellulite. Some Chinese and Indian women use boiled flowers and leaves mixed with herbal oil as a stimulant to hair growth. The flower's juice is used in black dye for the hair and mascara for eyebrows.

Horse chestnut extract (*Aesculus hippocastanum*)

This compound is used as a skin-conditioning agent. It also contains quercetin, so has anti-inflammatory and antibacterial properties.

Honey

Cleopatra knew a thing or two about beauty. Her fabled baths of milk and honey worked because honey is a humectant, which means that when honey is exposed to air, it draws in moisture. This may help to prevent scarring by keeping skin moist and help in the growth of new skin. Additionally, it helps to stop dressings becoming stuck to an open wound. For these reasons honey can be used as a moisturiser and skincare product. A common skin benefit from honey is related to minor acne treatment. Some varieties of honey are more active than others: Manuka honey from New Zealand has significant antibacterial properties associated with healing. Honey absorbs impurities from the pores on the skin, making it an ideal cleansing agent. Honey has a nourishing, bleaching and astringent effect on the skin. Japanese women have traditionally used honey for hand lotion. See also beeswax, royal jelly and propolis. There are more recipes in the later section. Here are some other uses:

○ For a hair conditioner mix 120 ml (4 fl oz) honey with 2 tablespoons olive oil. Work a small amount at a time through the hair until coated. Leave on for 30 minutes then shampoo well and rinse.
○ For a classically simple treat, try adding three or four tablespoons of honey to the bath water. You will enjoy a silky, fragrant bath.
○ For shiny hair, stir a teaspoon of honey into 1 litre (2 pints) of warm water. After shampooing and rinsing, pour the mixture through your hair. Do not rinse out.
○ To make a simple face mask, mix 3 tablespoons of oatmeal with 2 tablespoons clear honey. Apply to a clean face and relax for 15 about minutes. Rinse well with warm water, depositing the oats in a bin.
○ Mix 3 tablespoons of honey and a teaspoon of cinnamon powder. Apply this paste on to pimples before sleeping and wash it off the next morning with warm water. Repeat daily for two weeks. Some Chinese women use a paste made from crushed orange seeds and honey for pimples.
○ Honey, egg yolk and sweet almond oil is said to make a good hand softener.
○ For chapped lips and skin, mix 2 tablespoons of honey, the same of lemon juice and a tablespoon of eau de Cologne.

Indigo (*Indigofera tinctoria*)
Indigo is a plant that produces dark violet/blue dye. Asian countries such as India, China and Japan have used indigo as a dye for centuries. Indigo was also

known to many ancient civilisations. Used mainly as a textile dye, indigo is also incorporated into some henna hair dyes, to turn brown hair black.

Jasmine (*Jasmimum*)
Jasmine has been used because of its sweetly fragrant flowers for centuries, particularly in religious ceremonies in Asian and Mediterranean countries. Pure jasmine oil is very rare and expensive, with many petals needed to obtain the essential oil which is used in soaps, cosmetics and exotic perfumes. It is a warming oil, used to revitalise and stimulate the skin, reducing problems.

Jojoba oil (*Simmondsia chinensis*)
Jojoba oil is a liquid wax produced in the seed of the jojoba, a shrub native to the southern USA and Mexico. This is an excellent facial moisturiser. Jojoba is a good natural preservative for prolonging the shelf life of products made with essential oils. It is more stable than safflower or almond oil. It is very similar chemically to human face oil or sebum. Some might argue that its best claim to fame is that it has been accepted as a cosmetic substitute for sperm whale oil.

Kohl
Kohl is a mixture of soot and other ingredients used for thousands of years by Middle Eastern, North African and Asian men and women to darken the eyelids as well as mascara for the eyelashes. See the history chapter for more details. Some pretty nasty additions in the past caused problems, although the ancient Egyptians used it to protect the eyes from infections. Ingredients like sandalwood, castor oil and ghee are believed to have medicinal properties and are still used in Indian medicines.

Lady's Mantle (*Alchemilla vulgaris, A. mollis*)
I've only ever considered this plant for ground cover or a useful 'filler' for flower arranging, but lady's mantle has cosmetic uses going back for hundreds of years.

Infusions of the plant's leaves and flowers can be used for skin cleansing and facial steams. Make an infusion by steeping a couple of handfuls of leaves and/or flowers in a cup of boiling water for about 15 to 20 minutes. Cool, strain and use as required.

Lanolin
Lanolin is a greasy yellow substance obtained from sheep and other wool-bearing animals. It has many properties that keep the fleece in good condition, including waterproofing and antibiotic action. As a spinner, I have found that the lanolin present in unwashed fleece is a great hand softener. You get used to the sheepy smell! Crude grades of lanolin also contain wool alcohols, which some people are allergic to. The extract is insoluble in water, but forms an emulsion. Commercial, medical grade lanolin is used for chapped lips, hands and dry skin. The oil of Olay products apparently got their name originally from lanolin.

Lavender (*Lavandula*)
The ancient Greeks used lavender and called it nardus, or nard. This aromatic group of shrubby flowers are native to the poor soils of the Mediterranean, tropical Africa and India. I can't imagine a garden without lavender. We grow it along our pool side in France and the aromatic effect is magical on a hot day. The plant is grown commercially for the perfume industry and lavender oil has antiseptic, antibacterial and anti-inflammatory properties. It is much in demand as a massage oil and in aromatherapy because of its

harmonising effect on the emotions and also on the skin. A mild solution of lavender water can be sprayed on to reddened skin to soothe sunburn.

The active components in lavender are geraniol, cineole and coumarin. These have a strong cleansing and germicidal effect. In cosmetics lavender is good for dry or oily skins, for psoriasis, acne and eczema and is also said to be an excellent treatment for minor burns. Lavender oil should be kept out of reach of children at all times and should not be used during the first three months of pregnancy. It is used extensively to perfume soap, toilet water, cologne and perfume and is also used in bath products and stimulating facial steams.

LEMONS

Lemon oil
Lemon essential oil is pale yellow colour with the refreshing aroma of fresh fruit. Some lemon oil includes synthetic citral that, along with limonene, provides the lemony smell and oil from plants such as lemongrass. The oil is extracted by cold-pressing the fresh peel.

Limonoids are natural plant chemicals that are abundant in citrus fruit. Many plants used in traditional healing are rich in limonoids. They are currently being studied for a wide variety of therapeutic effects such as antiviral, antifungal and antibacterial qualities. Lemon oil is powerfully astringent and antiseptic. It should not be applied to the skin in dilutions greater than 5 per cent, to avoid skin irritation. Lemon oil is good for oily skin and has rejuvenating properties.

Lemon juice

When applied to hair, citric acid opens up the outer layer, also known as the cuticle. While the cuticle is open, it allows for a deeper penetration into the hair shaft and so may damage the hair. Here are some of the many uses of lemon juice in beauty treatments:

- Slices of fresh lemon can lighten freckles.
- Use as a hair rinse for blondes by diluting the juice of half a lemon diluted in 500 ml (17 fl oz) of water.
- Mix the juice of one lemon or two limes with some mild shampoo. Massage in and sit in the sun for 20 minutes before rinsing and conditioning.
- Using lemon in a face pack makes for a zingy effect. Try using with honey, cucumber, oats or yoghurt. See the recipe section for details.
- Make a massage cream from equal amounts of egg yolk, lemon juice and olive oil.
- Lemon is good at removing odours from the hands, for example after peeling onions or garlic. It is also a stain remover. For the hands, take the rind of the lemon after the juice has been squeezed out and rub the fingers and hands with the remaining pulp. If you are a gardener like me, stains can be removed from nails and skin by soaking your nails in water with lemon juice or lemon slices.
- Removing dark circles underneath the eyes and on the neck. Be very careful under the eyes! Adding lemon juice to a jar of cleansing pads might do the trick.

Macadamia nut oil (*Macadamia integrifolia*)

This oil comes from the pressed nuts of the macadamia tree. It is said to be the best carrier oil for the skin and is rich in palmitoleic acid, making it one of the best regenerative oils, replenishing lipids that delete with age. Macadamia oil is very protective, with a high absorption rate, and has been successfully used to heal scars, sunburn, minor wounds and other irritations. It is popular in massage and aromatheraphy.

Myrrh

This ancient oil was used by the Egyptians for incense in religious ceremomies, for skin diseases, facial concoctions and embalming because of its ability to preserve the flesh. Myrrh is still used in perfumery, cosmetics and massage. It is said to reduce wrinkles and preserve a youthful complexion, so is good for mature skin. It has a slightly cooling effect, so would be especially useful in a hot dry climate. It helps to balance the hydration of the skin, while removing toxins from skin tissue and promoting tissue repair on wounds, sores and ulcers.

Neem tree/Margosa tree (*Azadirachta indica*)

The bark of this tree produces an amber coloured gum. The leaves contain quercetin and valuable minerals and they have been used for hundreds of years to make antibacterial washes and poultices. Today, neem oil is used in face packs, soaps, applications for mild skin and nail disorders, mouth wash, hand cleaners for gardeners and hair products. The oil is also used for burning and purifying the air.

Nettle (*Urtica dioica*)

The common nettle is rich in calcium, iron, vitamin A and C and has long been used for medicinal purposes. It is said to stimulate hair growth, to treat dandruff and to soften fair hair, and is used in shampoos and facials. See the next section for hair use.

Oats (*Avena sativa*)
The medicinal qualities of oats derive from all parts of the plant, including the straw, green stems and leaves. Additionally, soaps, oat milk and other preparations can be made from them. Oats have often been used in baths to help skin conditions, have helped burns to heal and can reduce the effects of eczema. Although generally used as a useful compound in skin care, oats can also trigger skin problems in some people, so always test a small area of skin first. Being rich in silica, oats are also known to help renew bones, skin, nails, hair and other tissue. Oat extract is especially used in products that have a moisturizing and anti-ageing effect, as well as in products that are used to alleviate acne, pimples and to treat problem skin. See the recipe section for more ideas. Here are some tips:

○ For an oil-free bath soak, mix equal amounts of oatmeal and cornflour and put into an old foot from a pair of tights. Lower into the running water. Soak and enjoy. The tights keep the oats from blocking up the plughole.
○ Make a very simple face mask with 2 tablespoons of uncooked porridge oats and 1 to 2 tablespoons of plain yoghurt. Use while fresh.
○ As a cleanser for sensitive skin, mix 250 ml (½ pint) of warm water with 120 g (4 oz) of oatmeal and a tablespoon of honey. Gently massage into your skin, rinse with more warm water and pat dry.
○ Make a simple cleanser. Mix 3 tablespoons of oatmeal and 2 tablespoons of clear honey. Apply to a clean face and relax for 15 about minutes. Rinse well with warm water, depositing the oats in a bin.

Olive oil

Olive oil has been used in a range of skin preparations, soaps, massage and bath oils. Pure olive oil produces a hard soap that dries quickly, is mild and non-drying to the skin. I've been using the same bar for ages, so I can verify that it lasts a long time. The ancient Greeks and Romans used the oil, using a special scraper to take off the excess. Olive oil can be used to moisturise patches of dry spots and stretch marks. It also appears in lip balm, shampoo, hand lotions, massage oil and dandruff treatment. Soaking fingernails in warm olive oil will apparently soften cuticles and may help brittle nails become more resilient. It can be thickened with beeswax, agar (a thickening extract of red algae), xanthum or glycerine to make an ointment.

Orange (*Citrus sinensis, C. reticulate*)

Orange fruit and peel are used as an ingredient for skin-conditioning in cosmetic items for antioxidant, antimicrobial and anti-inflammatory properties. See citrus oils and lemons.

Palmarosa oil (*Cymbopogon martini*)

Also called rose geranium, palmarosa oil is extracted from a straw-coloured grass with fragrant leaves or blades. Harvested before flowering, this plant gives more oil after being dried. Palmarosa oil has a floral, faint rose-like smell and is pale yellow in colour. It is often blended with more expensive rose oil and is used in soaps, perfumes, massage oil and cosmetics. More surprisingly, it is also used to flavour tobacco. Palmarosa oil can help clear up infections and prevent scarring, when added to washing water. In creams and lotions it has a moisturising and hydrating effect. It is said to be useful on dry skin and in treating athlete's foot.

Patchouli (*P. cablin*)
This centuries-old perfume is heavy and strong. Essential oil is distilled from several species of this shrubby member of the mint family, but *P. cablin* is supposed to be the best. The plant comes from Asia and is now grown also extensively in West Africa and the Caribbean, where it has apparently been used as a hair conditioner for dreadlocks. It may also be an insect repellent.

Peanut oil (*Arachis hypogaea*)
The peanut, or groundnut, is a species of the legume family, native to South and Central America. Peanut oil is good for dry skin and is also nutritious. Peanut oil has a variety of industrial uses involving varnish, lubrication and nitroglycerine. Many cosmetics contain peanut oil. There is some concern that moisturisers that contain peanut oil may trigger further allergies in children with nut allergies. Peanut oil is present in a range of products from sunblock to toothpaste, including nappy rash and eczema creams. This is definitely something to bear in mind when dealing with allergies.

Petroleum Jelly
In the first part of the twentieth century, petrolatum, or petroleum jelly, was popular as a hair pomade and moustache wax, mixed with beeswax. Most petroleum jelly today is used in skin lotions and cosmetics. It is less expensive than glycerine but is not used in some products because it leaves a greasy feel to the skin. Many people prefer to avoid its use today.

Propolis
This is a resin collected by bees from trees and plants. When taken back to the hive it is mixed with

wax and used for a variety of protective as well as defensive purposes. Propolis has antibacterial, anti-fungal and anti-inflammatory properties and has been used by man for over 3000 years.

The resin is made of about 50 per cent resin, 30 per cent wax, 10 per cent essential oils and 5 per cent pollen. Propolis is used by the bees as a sticky filler and glue to protect the hive as a sterile environment. Over the last thirty years medical research has begun to uncover the secrets of propolis as a natural antibiotic. The substance can now be bought as a tincture to treat many ailments.

Pumpkin seed oil (*Cucurbita pepo*)
Made from the common pumpkin, this is said to be a highly nourishing oil that helps prevent excess moisture loss. Pumpkins are a really good vegetable to eat as well, packed full of goodies for the whole body. Pumpkin seeds contain fatty acids, protein and much more.

Rice bran wax (*Oryza sativa*)
Rice bran wax is the vegetable wax extracted from the bran oil of rice. This is used as an emollient, contains fatty acids and is the basis material for some exfoliation particles. Its use appears in a list of ingredients of a number of natural cosmetic products and as a substitute for carnauba oil.

Rosemary (*Rosmarinus officinalis*)
Rosemary is one of my favourite herbs. I was quite addicted to a rosemary shampoo some years ago, but it was discontinued. Rosemary oil contains camphor and eucalyptol, also found in eucalyptus and bay leaves. This aromatic oil is added to soaps, creams, perfumes and toilet water. It is used to darken hair,

and to condition all hair types. Try mixing it with shampoo to strengthen the hair. An infusion also makes an invigorating toner and astringent. Rosemary leaves added to a bath are very refreshing. Rosemary also contains soluble antioxidants.

Rose oil (*Rosa damascena, R. centifolia*)
The rose has a variety of uses and has been used for centuries by different civilisations for creating essential oils for perfume.

Rose oil, the essential oil extracted from the petals, can be rose otto (attar of roses), or rose absolute. The former is extracted through steam distillation, whereas rose absolutes are obtained using solvents. These are more commonly used in perfumes. Distilled rose oil is very valuable and still the most widely used essential oil in perfumery. It has been estimated that it takes about 4,000 kilograms (8,800 lb) of flower petals to make 1 kilogram (2 lb) of oil. Cheaper oil can be extracted by using solvents but these often contain synthetic additions. Palmarosa (see above) is sometimes added.

Rose otto is a dark, olive green colour and will form white crystals at room temperature. These disappear when the oil is warmed. It has a very strong smell and was the product much sought after in India, Persia and the Ottoman Empire. Most of it is now made in Bulgaria. It doesn't smell the same as fresh roses.

Rose absolute is a deep, reddy brown colour, with no crystals. The perfume is much more like fresh roses.

Rose-water
Rose-water is a by-product of rose oil production. It has softening, toning and healing properties and was

much in favour during Victorian times, to soothe the skin. It was also used for cleansing and for rinsing the hair. It finds its way into many recipes, both beautifying and culinary.

Royal jelly

This is the food fed to a potential queen bee larva. It is creamy white and very rich in protein and fatty acids. It is produced by the mouth glands of worker bees and used to feed developing young. All bee larvae are fed royal jelly for the first three days of development. Queen larvae are fed it during their entire larval development. Each queen needs only a teaspoon of royal jelly. As a health product, it is very expensive and almost tasteless. Only small quantities can be removed from the hives. It is mostly associated with human consumption for promoting energy and health and is considered by many to be a potent anti-oxidant. It appears in face creams and moisturisers as an anti-ageing ingredient.

Safflower oil (*Carthamus tinctorius*)

This is a moisturising oil with an exceptionally high amount of oleic acids. It can be soothing and is one of the first choices for skincare recipes requiring moisturising benefits. The flowers provide dyestuffs in shades of pink. When dried and mixed with French chalk it makes rouge. It is also used for medicinal and culinary applications.

Japanese geishas wore lipstick made of crushed safflower petals and also painted the eyebrows and eyelids with it.

Sea buckthorn oil (*Hippophae rhamnoides*)

This is extracted from sea buckthorn berries and produces an oil used to treat damaged skin, scar tissue, burns and wrinkles. It can be applied directly to the skin or mixed with other preparations to treat problematic skin conditions. Some mild staining of skin may occur, but this is apparently temporary and washes off easily. This oil is rich in essential fatty acids and carotenes.

Sea salt
High-quality sea salt is perfect for creating bath salts or body scrubs. They can be blended with dried herbs, flowers and essential oils. The mineral content of the Dead Sea, combined with the lack of pollen and other allergens, have great benefits to some patients with respiratory problems. People suffering from skin disorders also benefit, in two different ways. Firstly the reduction in harmful rays means that they can expose their skin to the sun for longer periods and secondly the salts in the water have been shown to help psoriasis patients. Year-round sun, dry air and low levels of pollution all help.

Some popular therapies are:

○ Climatotherapy and heliotherapy — that's sunbathing and taking the air
○ Thalassotherapy, or bathing in Dead Sea water
○ Balneotherapy, or treatment with black mineral mud.

Several varieties of Dead Sea salt are now available for treatments, so that you don't have to go there to benefit.

Sesame oil (*Sesamum indicum*)
Although much more commonly used as a salad dressing, this oil has been used since Babylonian times. Ancient Persians used it both as a food and for

its medicinal qualities. It has also been well known in China for around 5,000 years and is used in ayurvedic medicine in India.

Sesame oil has some natural sunscreen qualities, is rich in anti-inflammatory properties and is anti-bacterial on the skin. It is used to treat athlete's foot, psoriasis and dry skin ailments. It has been successfully used to kill head lice infestations. After exposure to wind or sun it will calm burning. Sesame oil is naturally active in vitamins A and E and essential proteins. Because of its relatively stable shelf life it is a good ingredient to include in body care products and natural cosmetics.

Shea butter (*Vitellaria paradoxa*)
This is obtained from the fruit of the African karite tree. It is traditionally used for a variety of skin problems such as eczema and dermatitis, to fade scars and discolouration and is widely used as a moisturiser and emollient. It is also found in conditioners for dry hair. As a sunscreen its effects are limited.

The butter is a slightly yellowy natural fat extracted by crushing and boiling the fruit of the tree. It is also edible.

Shilajit
Shilajit, found in the Himalayas, is believed to be the fossilised form of plants growing in prehistoric times. It is well known in ayurvedic medicine and is collected in lumps during summer months when the ice melts. It is presented in capsule form for human consumption. It is claimed that Shilajit is the most potent anti-ageing substance ever known to mankind, containing more than eighty-five minerals and fulvic

acid, a natural extract from ancient plant deposits, created seventy-five million years ago. There are claims that this restores electrical balance to damaged cells, neutralises toxins and can eliminate food poisoning within minutes.

Soapberry, soapnut (*Sapindus laurifolia, S. Mukorossi*) This natural detergent comes from a genus of up to twelve species of shrubs and small trees in the Sapindaceae family that are native to warm, temperate/tropical regions. Both common names refer to the use of the crushed seeds to make soap. They contain saponins and quercetin and are popular ingredients in ayurvedic shampoos and cleansers. They are also used as a treatment for eczema and psoriasis, and for removing freckles. Soapnuts have insecticidal properties and have been traditionally used for removing head lice.

Soapnut is found in cleansing lotions, shampoos and conditioners. Some other uses include:

○ Removing stains from hands.
○ When added to a facial made with milk powder and clay it provides delicate cleansing of the skin.
○ It can be added to salt body scrubs.
○ Add 1 teaspoon of soapnut extract to a cup of water to use as a hair wash or mild cleanser. It can also be combined with amla, neem and shikakai extract for a richer, antibacterial hair wash. Mix the herbs in water until dissolved. Keep refrigerated and use within four days.

Spearmint (*Mentha spicata*)
This commonly grown mint is used mainly for culinary purposes at home, but also has wide applications within cosmetics and perfumes. During the Middle

Ages, mint leaves were used in powdered form to whiten teeth. Menthol, from the essential oil of mint, appears in many cosmetics and some perfumes. Menthol and mint oil are also very popular in aromatherapy.

Spearmint is used to refresh and cool the skin in facials, bath products, toothpaste, mouthwash and hair oil. It is also found in air fresheners, combined with lavender or bergamot.

Sunflower oil (*Helianthus annuus*)
As well as helping to retain moisture, research suggests that sunflower oil may protect premature babies from infection. The oil is expressed from the seeds, to produce a light oil that is high in linoleic acid, vitamins and minerals.

Talcum powder
Talcum powder is produced from a magnesium trisilicate mineral called talc. In its natural form it may contain asbestos, a known human carcinogen. Since the 1970s all baby powders, body and facial powders have been asbestos-free. Cosmetic grade talcum powder has been used in baby powder for preventing nappy rash for generations. Recent research projects have suggested that there might be a small risk of developing ovarian cancer in women who use talcum powder regularly on genital areas. Other research has looked at the link between inhalation of industrial-grade talc and lung cancer.

Tamanu oil (*Calophyllum tacamahaca*)
This oil is extracted by a cold-pressed method from the whole nuts of the tamanu tree, native to Polynesia. Tamanu oil has the ability to heal damaged skin, including scarring, stretch marks, rashes, minor

cuts and abrasions. It can be used directly on the skin or mixed within formulations.

Thanaka (*Limonia acidissima and others*)
The wood of several different thanaka trees may be used to produce thanaka cream. This yellowy cosmetic paste is made from grinding the bark of the tree with a few drops of water. The light creamy paste is usually applied to the cheeks as round patches. For over 2,000 years this paste has been an essential part of the beauty routine of Myanmar women. It helps remove acne, promotes smooth skin and acts as a sunblock and apparently has a scent similar to sandalwood. Thanaka also gives a cooling sensation and has antifungal properties.

Tea tree oil (*Melaleuca alternifolia*)
Australian aboriginals used tea tree leaves for healing cuts, burns and infections. Tea tree oil is now most commonly used as an essential oil but is also an ingredient in creams, ointments, lotions, soaps and shampoos. It contains terpenoids, which have been found to have antiseptic and antifungal activity. It can be used to treat eczema, acne, athlete's foot, dandruff, fungal infections of the toenail and infestations of head lice. Some people have an allergic reaction to this oil as it also contains cineole, which can be an irritant to the skin. It should not be used undiluted unless tested first. As terpinoids are mild, the oil can soothe cuts, scratches, sunburn and cold sores. It can usually be applied as a single drop to minor injuries once or twice a day.

Turmeric (*Curcuma longa*)
This rhizome is a member of the ginger family. Turmeric is nature's internal cosmetic and an excellent natural antibiotic. Turmeric's antiseptic and healing

properties help counteract pimples, acne, boils and skin diseases. In India it is an inexpensive beauty aid. Smearing with turmeric paste cleans the skin.

Vetiver (*Chrysopogon zizanioides*)
This tropical scented grass from India has an earthy smell and amber colour. The oil, which has calming, therapeutic qualities, is extracted from the roots. It is popularly used for soaps, toiletries, moisturisers for dry skin and perfumes. It is used for blending in massage oils or for the bath, to combat exhaustion and skin complaints.

Violet (*Viola odorata*)
Violet oil is important in perfumery. The violet plant has long been cultivated for its use in medicines, cosmetics and perfume. The flowers are good for skin rashes and eczema. Decoctions from the flowers have been used as an eyebath and mouthwash. Sweet violets, either fresh or dried, are used in teas or baths for their soothing, astringent quality. Violets contain salicylic acid and are extremely high in vitamins A and C. Violet flower water is a traditional remedy facial tonic and aftershave. The leaves and flowers can be macerated in oil, strained and added to beeswax as a make-up remover. Violets are used in lip gloss, lotions and creams. The plant contains saponins. Chinese medicine uses violets to treat infectious skin conditions including boils. The colour of the flowers can be gathered by infusion and this has been used for eye shadow and tinted skin lotions. Interestingly, this infusion turns red when in contact with acid and green with alkali. Nature's answer to litmus paper!

Vinegar
Vinegar has many benefits for improving the skin, hair rinsing and foot odour problems. There are many

varieties, but cider vinegar seems to have many helpful properties, as well as a better smell than many others. See a later section.

○ Soak your feet in vinegar and water. It changes skin pH so that the fungus cannot grow. Soak for three evenings in a row.
○ Put ½ cup of vinegar into a bowl to soak your feet in before a pedicure. It softens your skin beautifully.
○ After-sun treatment: put vinegar in a spray bottle with water and spray on to sunburn, or mix a paste of bicarbonate of soda and apple cider vinegar and apply.
○ As a remedy for age spots, mix equal parts of onion juice and vinegar and use daily on the spots. This will take a few weeks to work, just like an expensive remedy from a shop, although you may smell a bit like a crisp bag!
○ Try white vinegar under arms and other areas of the body as a natural deodorant. It won't stop perspiration, but it will neutralise any odour.
○ Used as a hair rinse, vinegar neutralises the alkali left by shampoos. It will give your hair an all-out shine, and remove surplus soap. Add a tablespoon or two of vinegar to the final rinse. The smell doesn't linger.
○ When you have dyed your hair, rinse with warm water then dilute white vinegar with water for the final rinse. Use the water as cold as you can stand it. This seals your colour so it doesn't fade out quite so quickly.

Walnut (*Juglans regia*)
Walnut shells are included in some soap cosmetics and dental cleaners, along with apricot seeds. Walnut oil is said to have many benefits when healing wounds and

treating skin problems. Walnut oil is useful against fungal and parasitic infections, eczema and herpes and may help eliminate warts. When used in a massage blend it has great emollient qualities. Walnut oil presents good moisturising, anti-ageing and toning properties for all skin types. I seem to remember using a tanning lotion with walnut oil in my youth, obviously when I didn't mind looking like a bit of wood.

Wheat germ oil (*Triticum aestivum*)
This is a good source of vitamin E and an excellent oil for use on dry skin, although the strong smell might be a turn off. It is used in some mixes of massage oil. Eating wheat germ oil will probably be a better option for health because of the content of minerals, vitamins and fatty acids. Vitamin E promotes skin cell formation and is good for nourishing and rejuvenating mature, dehydrated skin, reducing scars and stretch marks and repairing sun-damaged skin. It has anti-inflammatory and antioxidant effects.

Witch hazel (*Hamamelis virginiana*)
Made from the leaves and twigs, witch hazel acts as an astringent and reduces inflammation.

Woad (*Isatis tinctoria*)
Woad, or glastum, is a plant producing a blue dye, and it is also used to dye hair. It is more colourfast in hair than indigo, but it does not create a deep blue-black. Woad was cultivated throughout Europe during ancient times, although historians now think that this was not the dye used by the Picts. This group got their name from the Romans (*Picti* means 'painted people') because of their habit of going into battle wearing only body paint or tattoos. Woad does not work well in this context.

Ylang-ylang
The fragrant essential oil is produced from the small flower of the cananga tree. The scent of ylang-ylang is rich with deep hints of jasmine. Used in aromatherapy, ylang-ylang is believed to correct sebum secretion in skin problems.

Zinc oxide
There had to be a Z, which is for zinc oxide, used to treat or prevent minor skin irritations such as burns, cuts and nappy rash. It is also used as a sunscreen. Our bodies need zinc to maintain healthy skin and one sign of zinc deficiency can be dry skin. Zinc helps to heal skin wounds. The best way to ensure that you have enough zinc is through a healthy diet.

Zinc oxide cream is mildly astringent and anti-inflammatory. It is also a natural insect repellent and sunscreen. In a mixture with small amounts of iron oxide, zinc oxide is called calamine, the basis of calamine lotion. Zinc can also relieve dandruff and is often found in shampoos. Some medical conditions may interact with zinc oxide cream and some chemical additives may cause reactions.

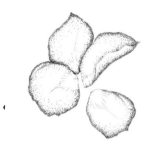

FACIAL
TREATMENTS

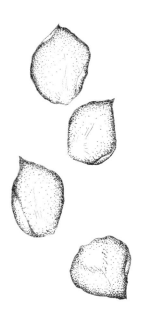

INDEX OF FACIAL TREATMENTS

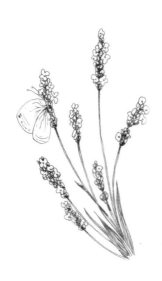

FACIAL STEAMS

Facial steams seem like a great idea if you are trying to avoid putting lots of products on to your skin. As a bit of a minimalist in the area of facials, moisturisers, skin packs etc they fit the bill entirely for me and can be great if you have any congestion or tension headaches.

Facial steams can help more than just overworked pores and glands. The warmth used for steaming helps to ease muscular and mental tension and to boost circulation, given that we have so many muscles in our faces. You shouldn't overdo the frequency, however, if you have dry skin. If your skin is dull or prone to blackheads this treatment is ideal.

Preparation involves tying long hair back out of the way and cleaning the face and neck with a light cleanser. Wash with pure soap and warm water, rinsing with tepid water. Pat dry gently.

Prepare the herbs by putting them in a medium-sized bowl and pouring over about 1 litre (2 pints) of boiling water over them. Next, lean over the bowl and place a clean towel over your head and the bowl so that the steam doesn't escape. Be careful not to get too close!

Relax (!) for about ten minutes. It doesn't sound very relaxing, but the steam will gradually start to relieve tension. This is best done away from any other family members, as the laughing and silly comments that ensue are not good for relaxation, even if laughing is good for you.

Remove the towel, wipe the face with a clean damp towel and dab with a freshener or toilet water. Stay inside for a while until your face cools down.
Here are some suggested combinations of herbs, although the choice is really up to you. You can just use one herb if you prefer.

Borage
Burnet
Chamomile flowers
Comfrey leaves.
Elderflowers
Fennel
Lady's mantle
Lavender
Lemon grass
Lime (linden) flowers
Marigold flowers
Nettle
Peppermint
Sage
Violets

SKIN REFRESHERS AND INFUSIONS

After cleansing or washing, a freshener of herbal infusion will act as a skin tonic. These can be made to suit all skin types. Those made with cider vinegar, raspberry vinegar or other fruits can be very drying, so should only be used on oily skin and not too often. There are herbs for all skin types. Here are some suggestions, although they are only a few of the many beneficial plants around.

Elderflower — for softening and lightening the skin
Lemon balm — for wrinkles
Lime (linden) flowers — for improving circulation
Marigold flowers — for skin with large pores or prone to pimples
Nettle — for firming the skin
Parsley — for fading freckles
Peppermint — for soothing the skin
Rose — for softening the skin
Rosemary — an astringent
Sage — for oily skin
Violets — to help clear blemishes

INFUSIONS
Infusions are easy to make — just like making a cup of tea. Just steep the herbs in 225 ml (8 fl oz) of boiling water until cool. Strain and use within 12 hours.

Here are some other tonics and infusions you might like to try.

Lady's mantle infusion
Use 1 tablespoon chopped leaves and flowers to 150 ml (5 fl oz) boiling water water. Leave to cool and strain.

Rose-water

The method is the same as above, but use strongly scented rose petals. You'll need about 225 g (8 oz) of petals in all. After bottling, store for a few days before use.

Marigold water

Put 25 g (1 oz) of marigold petals and 400ml (1 fl oz) in a pan and bring to the boil. Simmer for 30 minutes. Strain carefully and add another 25 g (1 oz) of petals to the liquid. Repeat the boiling and simmering and then strain again. Leave to cool and you should end up with about 300 ml ($1/2$ pint) of marigold water to store in a labelled, plastic bottle.

Nettle tea

Make a weak nettle tea as a face wash to firm up skin and remove excess oils. Nettle vinegar made with one part fresh nettle leaves to six parts cider vinegar makes a good astringent.

Peppermint infusion

Use 2 tablespoons of chopped peppermint leaves in 150 ml (5 fl oz) of boiling water. Use when strained and cooled for a soothing brew which is also good for mild sunburn.

Herb vinegar

This has the benefit of smelling as good as herbal water, but keeping for longer. Use cider vinegar or white vinegar at a push. Add 225 ml (8 fl oz) water to the same amount of vinegar. Heat until nearly boiling and then add dried herbs. Leave overnight to infuse before straining and bottling. Herbs to try include thyme, lavender, rosemary or violet. An alternative is to use a tablespoon of lemon balm with twice as much peppermint.

FACE MASKS, TONERS AND CLEANSERS

Most of these natural treatments can be made from ingredients you find in the kitchen, apart from the essential oils of course. Some are more unusual than others. I offer them for interest and suggest that any new ingredient is tested on the wrist before applying to the face, especially if you have sensitive skin.

Generally, dry skin can be helped by using the following herbs:

> Comfrey
> Fennel
> Lady's mantle
> Marigold
> Elderflower
> Salad burnet

Oily skin can take a bit of astringency, so these are good to try:

> Chamomile
> Sage
> Parsley
> Yarrow
> Peppermint

Most of us have combination skin types, so that makes life a bit more complicated.

CLEANSING OILS

As well as herbal infusions, you can make herbal oils to use as a cleanser. These are especially good for dry skin. Almond, sunflower and safflower oil are easy to use. You can use any one of the following to add to small jars of oil which you can label and leave covered as the herbs work their magic.

> Chamomile flowers
> Comfrey
> Elderflowers
> Lime (linden) flowers
> Nettle
> Peppermint
> Rosemary
> Violet

Alternatives are coconut oil or wheat germ oil. Coconut oil, which is solid at normal temperatures, needs heating to become usable. For this type of oil you need to simmer about 2 tablespoons of coconut oil in a pan with the herbs for 5 minutes before cooling and putting into a small jar with a close-fitting lid.

ROSE AND MARIGOLD MOISTURISER

This is a good moisturiser to use after you have had a face pack. See the section above for making your own rose-water and marigold water.

INGREDIENTS
   2 tablespoons glycerine
   2 tablespoons rose-water
   2 tablespoons marigold water

Method
The simplest way to do this is to use a clean screw-topped jar and mix it as if you were making salad dressing. Shake well until all the ingredients are mixed. Shake just before using. Apply with fingers or cotton wool sparingly. Wipe off with tissue.

LEMON, MILK AND ALMOND SCRUB

Use equal amounts of finely grated lemon rind and powdered milk with 2 parts ground almonds. Mix with lemon juice for a zingy scrub.

STRAWBERRY AND HONEY FACE SCRUB

Ingredients
> medium-sized strawberries
> 60 g (2 oz) oatmeal, uncooked
> 2 teaspoons green tea
> 3 teaspoons honey

Method
Wash and hull the strawberries. Blend the oatmeal, strawberries, green tea and honey. Apply a small amount to the skin, avoiding the eyes and using fingertips and circular motions to work into the skin. Repeat until the face and neck are covered. Rinse completely, using lukewarm water. Store the remaining scrub in a covered container in the fridge for up to a week.

ROSE OIL AND HONEY MASK

Ingredients
> 2 tablespoons honey
> 2 tablespoons sweet almond oil
> 5 drops essential oil of rose

Method
Mix the honey and oils. Massage on to the face and neck with fingertips. Relax for 15 minutes, then rinse off with lukewarm water.

GREEN HONEY MASK

Maybe this is better for Halloween! Alternatively you could try this with a friend and see who makes the best scary face. I'm afraid it will stay in the realms of theory for me. I'd rather eat the spinach, ginger and banana and hope that they benefit more than just my face.

Ingredients
- 1 small packet fresh spinach, washed
- 2 tablespoons fresh mint
- 1 teaspoon fresh ginger, crushed
- 3 tablespoons honey
- 1 ripe banana
- 2 egg whites

Method
Blend the spinach, mint and ginger together. Add the honey and banana and blend until you have a liquid consistency. Add the egg whites and mix thoroughly. Apply a small amount to the entire face and neck, except the eyes. Allow to remain on the skin for 15–20 minutes while you take pictures to scare people with. Rinse and apply moisturiser.

APPLE TONER

INGREDIENTS
- 1 tablespoon honey
- 1 apple, peeled and cored

Method
In a blender, purée the honey and apple. Smooth over the face and leave on for 15 minutes. Rinse with cool water.

LIME JUICE TONER

Cut a lime into slices and rub on the face slowly
2–3 times. Leave for about 5 minutes, then wash with
cool water. Repeat 3 times a week, if you can
stand it.

CUCUMBER AND HONEY TONER

Purée half a cucumber in a blender and drain away
the liquid. Add a teaspoon of honey and mix well.
Apply to the face and neck area with cotton wool.
Leave to dry and then rinse clean.

MOISTURE MASK, CLEOPATRA STYLE

Mix 2 tablespoons of honey with 2 teaspoons of milk.
Smooth over the face and throat. Leave for 10
minutes before rinsing off with warm water.

FIRMING FACE MASK

Ingredients

   1 tablespoon honey
   1 egg white
   1 teaspoon glycerine
   2 tablespoons cornflour (approx)

Method

Whisk together all ingredients and enough cornflour
to form a paste. Smooth over the face and throat.
Leave on for 10 minutes while you relax, before
rinsing off with lukewarm water.

HAWAIIAN FACIAL

Using green tea bags would make this simpler but, if not, infuse the green tea in less than half a cup of boiling water.

Ingredients (2 treatments)
   $^1/_2$ ripe papaya
   150 g (5 oz) fresh pineapple, diced
   2 tablespoons green tea
   2 tablespoons honey

Method
While this is cooling, peel the papaya and remove the seeds. Blend the papaya and pineapple until pureed. Combine the honey with the fruit and add the cooled green tea (don't make it too runny). Mix well. Apply to the face with your fingertips and rest for 10–15 minutes. Remove completely with tepid water and tissues. Store the surplus in a covered container in the fridge for up to a week.

AVOCADO AND CUCUMBER FACE MASK

Avocado on its own is a great help if your problem is dry skin. Mash half a ripe avocado and apply it gently on to the dry areas on your skin. Rinse off after 15 minutes.

Ingredients
   $^1/_4$ cucumber, peeled and chopped
   $^1/_2$ avocado
   1 tablespoon fresh lemon juice
   3 tablespoons finely powdered oats
   3 tablespoons of water
   1 teaspoon honey

few drops of essential oils (optional)

8–9 tablespoons green clay or kaolin

Method

Purée the cucumber and avocado flesh in a food processor with the water and lemon juice until smooth. Add the oats, honey and essential oils. Pour the mix into a bowl and then whisk in the clay. Apply to the face and neck and leave on for 20–30 minutes. Rinse off with warm water then use a toner and moisturiser.

PUMPKIN FACE MASK

Pumpkins are full of betacarotene and vitamin A, making them especially nourishing for your skin. This sounds like another ideal recipe to try at Halloween time. You might not even need to buy a mask. I think I'd rather stick to eating the pumpkins in some delicious soup.

Ingredients

1 miniature pumpkin, or portion of a larger one

4 pineapple chunks

1 tablespoon finely powdered oats

1 tablespoon finely powdered almonds

1 teaspoon milk

1 teaspoon honey

1 teaspoon olive oil

2 drops rose geranium essential oil

Method

1. Use a sharp knife to core the pumpkin and slice on a cutting board. Cut about 6–8 pieces.

2. Place pumpkin pieces (including seeds) in a microwave-safe dish with about 1/2 cup of water.

Microwave for about 2 minutes until the flesh is soft. Allow to cool.

3. Cut the peel off and place the pumpkin flesh and seeds into a food processor with the pineapple and blend until smooth.

4. Add the oats, almonds, milk and honey, processing after each addition. Add the oil and essential oil and stir. The texture should be fairly rich and smooth, with just a slight graininess.

To use, apply to cleaned and toned face and neck skin. Rest for 15 minutes. Rinse well with warm water and follow with a moisturiser.

CUCUMBER FACE MASK FOR SENSITIVE SKIN

Ingredients

    1 large cucumber, peeled and deseeded

    1 tablespoon whipping cream

    $1/2$ tablespoon clear honey

    about 8 teaspoons finely powdered oats

Method

1. Place the peeled and seeded cucumber in a blender and process until liquefied.

2. Add the whipping cream and honey and process until smooth. Add the oats and process further until a paste-like mixture is formed. Add more oats if the cucumber was very watery.

3. Smooth a thick layer over clean skin and rest for 15 minutes. Rinse with warm water and apply a moisturiser.

DEEP HONEY AND OATMEAL CLEANSER

Ingredients

- 1 tablespoon honey
- 1 tablespoon oatmeal
- 2 slices cucumbers

Method

Mix the honey and oatmeal together till thick. Adjust the proportions if necessary. Apply as a face-pack and place the cucumber on your eyes. Rest for half an hour then wash off.

OATMEAL AND VINEGAR OR OIL CLEANSER

This is a recipe made entirely from ingredients from the store cupboard. The choice of olive oil or vinegar for mixing is up to you and your skin type. Olive oil is best for normal to dry skin and vinegar if your skin tends to be on the greasy side. Don't use malt vinegar, however, which is chemically produced and won't smell nice, apart from possibly making your skin smart. Cider vinegar or any mild fruit vinegar would be best. You don't need much, anyway. It will keep for up to three months, so you could increase the proportions, but I think it is best to make just enough for one application.

Ingredients

- 1 tablespoon finely ground oats
- 1 tablespoon wheat bran
- 1 tablespoon honey
- olive oil or cider vinegar to form a paste

Method

Mix the oatmeal, wheat bran and honey together in a bowl. Add enough olive oil or cider vinegar to form a paste. Rinse your face with warm water, apply the cleanser and massage it gently into the skin. Rinse with warm water then splash your face with cold water.

LADY'S MANTLE FACE PACK

Ingredients

- 3 tablespoons wheat germ
- 1 tablespoon honey
- 2 tablespoons lady's mantle infusion

Method

For a stimulating face pack for normal skin, mix the ingredients thoroughly and apply to the face. Leave for 20 minutes before removing with tepid water.

HEMP SEED FACE POLISH WITH GREEN TEA
(FOR MEN)

Hemp seed flour contributes a smooth exfoliating texture with the benefits of essential fatty acids. Green tea is a good antioxidant and oat flour a soothing cleanser. Chickpea flour can be used instead, for convenience. You can vary or omit some of the essential oils for ease and economy.

Ingredients

- 150 g (5 oz) oat flour
- 150 g (5 oz) hempseed flour (or chickpea flour)
- 2 green tea bags
- 15 drops lime essential oil
- 5 drops cypress essential oil

5 drops lavender essential oil
5 drops juniper berry essential oil

Method
Place the oat flour and hemp seed flour in a clean bowl. Break open the green tea bags and add to the flours. Mix well. Add the essential oils, one by one, stirring after each.

Transfer to a clean air-tight container. Leave the mixture for 3–5 days before using.

To use, scoop a clean spoonful of the mixture into the palm of your hand. Mix with enough water or herbal tea to make a smooth paste. Massage gently over face and neck. Rinse well.

OAT, LEMON AND GINGER FACIAL

The essential oils are cleansing and astringent while the oats are soothing and gentle.

Ingredients
2 tablespoons ground oats
1 tablespoon buttermilk (or skimmed milk)
1 egg white
1 drop ginger essential oil
1 drop lemon essential oil

Method
Combine the buttermilk and egg white. Stir vigorously. Add to the oats and stir until a smooth paste forms. If the mixture is too runny, add a few more oats to absorb some of the liquid. Add the essential oils and stir.

To use, smooth a layer of the mask over the face and neck, avoiding the eyes. Rest for 10–15 minutes. Rinse well with warm water and pat face and neck dry. Follow with toner and moisturizer.

HONEY, ALMOND AND LEMON CLEANSER

Ingredients
- 1 tablespoon honey
- 2 tablespoons finely ground almonds
- $1/2$ teaspoon lemon juice

Method
Mix all the ingredients and dab gently onto the face. Rinse off with warm water.

TURMERIC AND FRESH LIME JUICE PASTE

Citrus oils can do a lot of good if you have oily skin as they kill bacteria and dry up excess oil. Make a paste of turmeric powder with fresh lime juice and apply. This will need very careful washing off, otherwise you might look jaundiced.

EGG AND LEMON CLEANSER

Squeeze half a lemon and mix the juice with one beaten egg white. Apply on your face and leave for as long as possible. Wash your face with warm water.

LEMON AND CUCUMBER CLEANSER
(FOR OILY SKIN)

Apply equal amounts of lemon and cucumber juice on the face. Leave for 15 minutes and wash off.

OTHER TREATMENTS AND BALMS

EYE COMPRESSES

Obviously extreme care must be taken with eyes, but these measures may help you relax, brighten tired eyes and reduce puffiness. Avoid irritation by putting a layer or two of clean lint soaked in the infusion to the eyelids. After about ten minutes, remove and dap the eyes with fresh cold water. You could use separate infusions of the following:

> Chamomile
> Fennel
> Eyebright
> Elderflower

I've heard of people using spent herbal tea bags when cooled as well. The other old favourite is to apply slices of cucumber to the eyes while having a soak in the bath.

HONEY LIP BALM

This might be a nice present for friends, as the amount you make would take ages to use, or you could halve the quantities. Be very careful with hot beeswax.

Ingredients
    225 ml (8 fl oz) sweet almond oil
    115 g (4 oz) beeswax
    2 tablespoons honey

Method
Place the almond oil and beeswax in a microwave-safe bowl or in a bowl over a pan of hot water.

Microwave for about half a minute, until the mixture melts. Whisk the honey into the wax. When cool, pour into small containers with lids. Apply to lips as a moisturiser or on top of lipstick for extra shine.

BANANA BALM

Bananas offer a fruity remedy for dry skin or scaly skin. Mash one or two ripe bananas and apply to dry or scaly areas on your skin. Wait about ten minutes before rinsing off. This is a cleanser and moisturiser in one and suits all skin types, especially dry. The essential oil is optional.

Ingredients
  1/2 fresh banana
  1 teaspoon honey, slightly warmed
  1 tablespoon fresh whipping cream, lightly warmed
  about 1 tablespoon fine oatmeal
  few drops essential oil (optional)

Method
Mash the banana to a creamy pulp. Warm the honey and whipping cream in a microwave for about 15 seconds. Stir well, then add to the banana pulp. Add the oats and essential oil and stir again. To use massage over dampened skin using gentle, sweeping, upward motions. Rinse well and follow with a toner and moisturiser.

CUCUMBER AND HONEY EYE NOURISHER

Always be careful when applying new ingredients to the face, especially on the delicate skin under the eyes. Avoid getting any of the ingredients into your eyes.

This recipe should reduce puffiness, cool and refresh the contour under the eyes.

Ingredients
- $1/2$ teaspoon chamomile tea
- 1 teaspoon cucumber, peeled with seeds removed
- $1/2$ tablespoon aloe vera gel
- $1/2$ teaspoon honey

Method
Infuse the chamomile tea in a small amount of boiling water (about an egg cupful). While this cools blend the cucumber, aloe vera and honey. Add the cooled camomile tea and mix thoroughly. Chill the cream before applying gently under the eyes. Store the surplus in a covered dish in the fridge for up to a week.

SPOT TREATMENTS

There seem to be hundreds of 'remedies' for pimples around, ranging from simple applications of herbs to very expensive ointments and creams. The most obvious solution seems to be to eat well and sleep well, but all sorts of other factors, sometimes unavoidable, affect our skin. These may result in conditions requiring professional help, so this section is not meant to replace that advice. Otherwise, there may be a recipe for disaster! Some of these solutions sound more like a medieval witch's brew or how to treat someone you don't like very much. That said, many of the ingredients suggested in the following list contain proven beneficial compounds that have been used in different cultures for generations.

- Apply 3 tablespoons of honey and one teaspoon of cinnamon powder paste to pimples before sleeping. Wash off next morning with warm water. Repeat nightly for 2 weeks.
- Grind nutmeg with fresh milk and apply on affected area.
- Apply equal amounts of lemon juice and cinnamon powder.
- Regularly rub fresh garlic on to spots, which will disappear quickly, just like your friends.
- Mix equal amounts of groundnut oil with fresh lime juice.
- Apply fresh mint juice over the face every night for the treatment of pimples.
- Apply a paste of fresh fenugreek leaves every night for 10—15 minutes and wash off with warm water.
- Apply raw papaya juice.
- Mix lime juice and rose water in equal portions to the affected area. Wash off after 20—30 minutes with lukewarm water.
- Apply ripe tomato pulp on to pimples and keep for up to an hour before washing.
- Apply grated potatoes as a poultice to treat skin blemishes.
- Make a paste of sandalwood with rose-water. Wash off after 20—30 minutes.
- Make a paste with ground radish seeds or sesame seeds and water.
- Make a paste of turmeric powder in mint juice. Leave on for about 25 minutes.
- Make a paste of neem leaves with turmeric powder and leave for 25 minutes.
- Make a paste from dried basil, mint juice and lemon juice.

PAPAYA PAMPERING

Papaya can give back the natural glow to lacklustre skin. Mash 115 g (4 oz) ripe papaya and cover the area for treatment. Leave on for about 15 minutes and then rinse for vibrant, fresh flesh.

GIVING THE ELBOW

As a child I always had very dry elbows. I don't know why, but they bothered other people more than me. Perhaps it was because they are also bony and pointed! Dry, elbows don't look attractive. You can exfoliate them with fresh pineapple. Rub some on to your elbows and rinse off after 15 minutes. Apply moisturiser to finish off.

HOME-MADE BODY GLITTER

Aloe vera gel is an excellent base for body glitter. Put a small amount into a clean jar, and mix in fine cosmetic glitter until you get the desired consistency.

SALT FACIAL

I think this will appeal to men rather than women, somehow. For a stimulating facial mix equal parts of sea salt and olive oil. Gently massage in with long upward strokes. Remove and wash with mild soap and warm water.

BODY SUGARING

This was used by the ancient Egyptians, or so I've heard. Body sugaring is a method for removing body hair that is an alternative to waxing or shaving. I have included it as an interesting alternative, but am not inclined to try this at home! As with waxing, there will be pain involved and heat, so it isn't everyone's cup of tea. I'm assured that it is less painful than waxing, but I'm afraid I'm not going to be a guinea pig for this one. I have painful memories of waxing while drinking wine in the past, but we won't go into that now.

The principle involves making a ball of sugary substance and cooling it, before applying to strips of cloth. Then, what a rip off! Proceed with extreme caution, if you must, and try out a small area of leg or arm first.

You will need a sugar thermometer and some strips of cotton fabric.

Ingredients
    450 g (1 lb) sugar
    8 tablespoons lemon juice
    8 tablespoons water

Method
1. Combine the ingredients in a heavy saucepan, and heat slowly. Watch the mixture very carefully so that it doesn't boil over. Heat the mixture to 130°C (250°F) on the thermometer.
2. Remove from the heat and let it cool enough to pour into a bowl or jar. This jar will be reheated in the future. Rip clean cotton fabric into strips.
3. Let the mixture cool so that it won't burn your skin. Test the mixture on the back of your hand.
4. Using a pallet knife or lolly stick, spread the cooled sugar on to your skin. Cover with the cloth strips, let it set for a few minutes and then rip off quickly. Ow!

5. You can reheat the mixture to a warm (but not hot!) temperature and reuse. Reheating will thicken the paste.

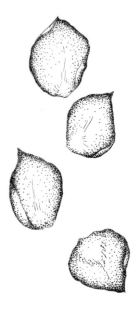

HANDS
AND
FEET

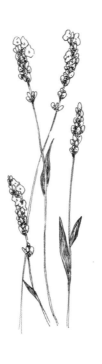

HANDS AND FEET

Hands and feet often get lumped together for treatment, although feet get far greater misuse than hands in general, although they too suffer neglect. I'm afraid my hands get a pounding in the garden when I forget to put the gloves on. There's something good about getting your hands in the soil from time to time, but the stains and rough skin can be a bit of a pain. Most of us spend time on face and hair but don't think too much about the way that our hands look, although after faces they are the most expressive part of our bodies. As for feet, would anyone want to be a podiatrist or a chiropodist? Come to that, who'd be a dentist either!

HAND TREATMENTS

Natural treatments involve applying few or no chemical products to your nails. Nail polishes and removers are usually made from harsh chemical products. The best way of keeping good strong nails is to make sure that your diet provides plenty of calcium, minerals and vitamins and includes fresh fruit and vegetables. As for false nails, I still wince when I remember the state of my friend's nails after she had her nail extensions removed. She had to grow them out because the glue destroyed the surface. Yuck!

I also remember as a child my mum using a polish for her nails that she applied from a small tin. I've just asked her what it was made from and she produced the original tin! It was called the Amami nail polishing stone. Apart from several offers to buy a vintage tin and stone on eBay, I found no other relevant information. My mum says she still takes her tin everywhere with her. It gives a shiny, slightly pink appearance to the nails.

NATURAL MANICURE

Here's how to naturally pamper your paws.
- Soak them in a bowl of warm water for two or three minutes and pat them dry.
- Then apply moisturiser or hand cream, working the moisturiser into the base of each nail.
- Using a soft cotton flannel or cuticle tool, gently push back the cuticles.
- Trim your nails and remove any jagged edges.
- Massage a little more moisturiser into your hands and fingers, working into the palm of your hand and up your wrist. This is nicer if you can

persuade someone else to massage your hands while you lie back and relax.
⟲ Buff your nails gently with the flannel cloth.

APRICOT, LEMON AND SUGAR HAND TREATMENT

Apricot oil is a good moisturiser. The sugar and lemon act to exfoliate and leave clean, soft hands.

Mix 115 g (4 oz) granulated sugar with a few tablespoons of apricot oil and the juice of $\frac{1}{2}$ a lemon or lime. Rub the mixture onto the hands and rinse with warm water. Apply hand cream afterwards.

NAIL AND HAND WHITENING TREATMENT

Lemon is good at removing odours from the hands, for example after peeling onions or garlic. It is also a stain remover. For the hands, take the rind of the lemon after the juice has been squeezed out and rub the fingers and hands with the remaining pulp.

If you are like me and forget to put gloves on when gardening, stains can be removed form nails and skin by soaking your nails in water with lemon juice or lemon slices. The lemon acts as an astringent and will take away stains.

As a point of interest, I also came across a suggestion that using lemon juice on nails three times a day prevents them from cracking or splitting.

HAND MOISTURISER

Ingredients

    2 tablespoons fine oatmeal
    1 tablespoon lady's mantle infusion (see A to Z section)
    1 teaspoon avocado oil
    1 teaspoon lemon juice
    1 teaspoon glycerine

Method

Mix all of the ingredients to form a smooth paste.
Apply to the hands and leave on for about 30 minutes
before washing off and moisturising.

HAND CREAM

If you have the equipment, time and inclination, you
might like to try this recipe.

Ingredients

    2 teaspoons beeswax
    1 teaspoon cocoa butter
    50 ml (2 fl oz) sunflower or almond oil

Method

Melt the wax and cocoa butter together in a bowl
over a pan of hot water. Add the oil and essential
oils to suit. You could use lavender, rosemary or
sandalwood (10 drops or so) and half this amount of
lemon oil. Pour the mix into a jar to cool. This is best
applied to the hands and nails at night so that the oils
can do their work.

SMOOTHING HAND AND ELBOW LOTION

Ingredients
1 teaspoon honey
1 teaspoon vegetable oil
1/4 teaspoon lemon juice

Method
Mix all the ingredients together. Rub into hands, elbows, heels and any other areas of dry skin. Leave on 10 minutes. Rinse off with warm water.

REMOVING SPLINTERS

Mix a little water with 1/2 teaspoon of bicarbonate of soda to form a paste. Apply this to a splinter and cover it with a plaster for a couple of hours. The soda should draw out the splinter, which can then be easily removed, along with any toxins, and solve the problem.

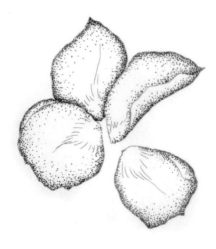

FOOT TREATMENTS

HONEY AND MINT FEET TREAT

This sounds perfect for restoring the circulation after a long day on the go. It moisturises and softens tired, aching feet.

Ingredients

- 4 teaspoons grated beeswax
- 4 tablespoons aloe vera gel
- 2 teaspoons honey
- 2 teaspoons freshly chopped mint, optional
- 6 drops peppermint essential oil
- 2 drops arnica oil
- 2 drops camphor oil
- 2 drops eucalyptus oil

Method

Melt the beeswax in a microwave and combine with the aloe vera and honey. Add the mint and oils, stirring until completely mixed. Apply after a bath or shower to the feet and toes. Store the remaining mixture in a cool place.

LIME AND GINGER SALT SCRUB FOR FEET AND ELBOWS

Dry or scaly skin can be rubbed with the peel of a lemon or lime. Rough elbows can be softened by rubbing the area with the cut side of a lemon or lime. This recipe combines other ingredients for special pampering.

Ingredients

1 teaspoon sea salt	1 grated lime rind
1 teaspoon camellia oil	1 teaspoon shredded root ginger

Method

Mix the ingredients together and scrub on to wet heels, feet, knees and elbows in gentle, circular motions.

FOOT CREAM

Use the recipe and method described for hand cream, but add 10 drops of each rosemary oil for circulation, 10 of lemon oil for refreshing tired feet and 5 drops of sage oil as a mild antiperspirant. Store in a jar until required.

ESSENTIAL FOOT BATH

You don't have to have a foot spa to enjoy a bit of foot massage and pampering. Just fill a bowl with warm water and add 6–10 drops of rosemary, sage, lemon, cypress, thyme or juniper oil. If you have them, put a few marbles into the bowl to help massage your feet. Relax and soak for about 20 minutes, then rub your soles and heels with a pumice stone. Pat dry and massage with the foot cream.

BICARB FOOT SOAK

Another way to put life and harmony back into tired, smelly feet is to soak them in a bowl of hot water with 4 tablespoons of bicarbonate of soda. Bliss! The soaking will also soften hard skin, which you can remove with a pumice stone.

PEDICURE PAMPERING

Put 115 ml (4 fl oz) of cider vinegar into a bowl of warm water and soak your feet before a pedicure. It softens the skin beautifully.

TREATMENTS AGAINST CORNS

Corns are usually caused by ill-fitting footwear or pressure on the toes. The best treatment is to avoid the pressure and avoid wearing shoes that rub. You can remove some of the thickened skin of corns and calluses by rubbing gently with a pumice stone while in the bath. Do this regularly and apply a soothing moisturising cream afterwards. Essential oils such as lemon, lavender, tea tree and peppermint are useful additions. Seek specialist advice if the problem recurs.

These are some less common suggested treatments, which I have never had cause to try, never having had a corn. Perhaps all those sensible shoes chosen for me when I was young have paid off!

- Cut a small onion in half and put the pieces in vinegar to stand for a couple of hours. Before going to bed place an onion half on each corn and tie it to your foot. In the morning scrape the softened corn. If necessary repeat the procedure several nights. This sounds like a recipe for disaster if sharing the bed with a partner who doesn't enjoy the smell of pickled onions as a night-time perfume!
- Apply undiluted lemon oil, several times a day.
- Apply tea tree and lavender massage oil to soften and soothe the skin.

FOOT ODOUR EATER

Feet are covered in sweat glands, so it's not surprising that they smell so much at times. Sometimes washing feet in the shower is just not enough. Soap with tea tree can help as it is an antibacterial, although shoes may also need deodorising. Use bicarbonate of soda as a substitute for talcum powder after washing your feet. Natural fibres are always best for feet, so cotton socks and leather shoes are preferable. If you don't wear socks the shoes will need separate treatment. Cotton shoe liners will help unless the shoes are sandal style, with open toes. Some shoes, for example, trainers and rubber flip flops can be washed in hot soapy water to get rid of the pong.

TOE NAIL FUNGUS

You might try using one part vinegar to one part warm water to soak your feet. Put a few drops of white vinegar on the nail several times a day for best results.

SCENTED FOOT MASSAGE

An aromatic massage oil containing peppermint and cypress oils can help to reduce perspiration. Add 8 drops cypress oil and 2 drops peppermint oil to 25 ml (1 fl oz) sweet almond oil and massage into your feet night and morning.

NATURAL TREATMENTS FOR ATHLETE'S FOOT

Keeping your feet clean and dry is essential. Avoid sharing towels as this can spread the infection. Seek proper advice if the problem persists. Here are some suggestions:

- Add five to six drops tea tree, lavender, peppermint or patchouli oil in a foot wash.
- Use a herbal footbath containing herbs such as rosemary, mustard seed, myrrh, peppermint or ginger.
- Apply calendula ointment on to clean, dry skin between the toes.
- Use talc containing lavender and/or peppermint.
- High-strength garlic capsules can also allegedly help beat the infection.

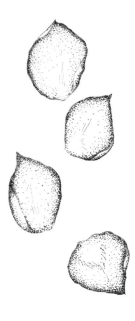

HAIR TREATMENTS WITH NATURAL INGREDIENTS

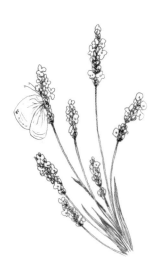

HAIR TREATMENTS

Hair should be your crowning glory, but there are times when we are all out of condition for one reason or another, and lacklustre hair is one outward and very obvious sign. There may be several reasons for this, such as:

- over-exposure to the sun
- polluted atmosphere that dries the hair
- excessive use of drying with intense heat, hair straighteners and heated rollers
- central heating and air-conditioning
- nutritional deficiencies
- lack of sleep
- hormonal changes in pregnancy and menopause
- use of artificial hair dyes and perming etc
- illness or shock

If you are experiencing serious symptoms such as excessive hair loss or severe dandruff seek professional advice. The information provided here is not meant to be a substitute.

HENNA TREATMENT AND DYEING

Henna is used by millions of women as a hair dye, conditioner and tonic. I have to come clean and say that I have never dyed my hair. I tried using a henna shampoo once, many years ago, but because my hair is very dark it made no difference. It probably didn't have much henna in it either. After that I've never bothered again, because I don't mind having grey hairs and think that they can look a lot better than roots of natural colour growing through as the hair grows and the dye fades.

WORDS OF CAUTION

Having seen the bizarre results that commercial dyes can give I think I'd rather leave it to experts, but even then things can go awry, as I remember from student days when my friend had to have her long, black hair cut very short after a bad dye day at the hairdressers.

TRIAL, NOT ERROR

Some essential advice is to use the hairs from a hairbrush to experiment on, if you are determined to go ahead. Try the mixture you are planning to use on these hairs first. Many henna dyes contain chemical additions in the form of metals, which will give different results from those expected. If you have previously dyed your hair with a chemical dye, the residue in the hair may also make a difference to the result.

Using henna to dye and condition your hair needs a long commitment, because you can't use a commercial dye over the top without risking an unwanted reaction.

Henna can take up to nine months or a year for the colouring to disappear. The sun may fade it to a lighter shade, but the hair will maintain its colouring for a long time. While the colouring remains, you will need to henna your hair every month or six weeks to maintain the conditioning.

Henna doesn't lighten the hair, so if you have dark hair it won't necessarily give the desired effect, but henna can provide burgundy highlights to dark hair. Each time you use henna the colour is likely to become deeper, so I might have had some success if I had persevered, but I'm not a risk taker when it comes to my appearance!

HOW MUCH POWDER?

Apparently, 100 g (3^1/$_2$ oz)of henna will dye a head of hair 30 cm (12 in) long, so you'll need to adjust the amount, depending on the length of your hair. Opened packets of henna need to be closed securely to prevent deterioration.

1. Put the henna into a plastic bowl with lukewarm water and/or lemon juice (half and half) to form a paste. Lemon juice will relax the hair. Stir until smooth. Leave, covered for at least two hours before using.

2. Wearing rubber gloves, apply the henna to your hair. Be careful of towels, clothes and furnishings. Apply from the roots to the tips. Cover with a plastic shower cap or plastic wrap and an old towel that you can use just for henna treatments. Henna stains, so protect your neck, ears and forehead with tissues or cotton wool, tucked into the cap, or petroleum jelly.

3. Leave for at least two hours. Hair types vary. Some will colour in 45 minutes whereas others take up to eight hours. The time spent beforehand on the hairbrush trial should help you to decide.

4. Rinse *thoroughly* until the water is absolutely clear. This is best done over a sink, unless you want rivulets of henna all over you! Any henna left in the hair will stain your bedding. Apply a conditioner to damp hair before combing and drying.

HENNA AND AMLA COLOUR

If you don't want to take the plunge entirely, this method might be for you. It is reported to take three or four weekly applications before the hair darkens to a burgundy colour. Follow the instructions regarding rubber gloves and stains above.

1. Mix 50 g (2 oz) of Henna extract, 10 g (1/3 oz) of amla extract with some tea water. Leave overnight in a plastic container.

2. Apply to the hair and leave on for at least two hours. Wash off and rinse thoroughly.

HENNA AND INDIGO DYES

Using both henna and indigo can result in black, purplish black or burgundy-black hair. The shade depends upon original hair colouring and the mixture used. There is no such thing as black henna, so any product that claims to be so is probably a mixture and may contain chemical additives. Always use 100 per cent pure quality henna powder. The depth of colour is dependant on the amount of indigo used.

Wear gloves and follow the test guidelines above. It sounds like a job for two people to me.

One-step method
Henna and Indigo application can be done in either a two-step or one-step process.

1. Prepare your henna paste as above. In a separate bowl mix indigo with warm water and leave to rest for 15 minutes before combining the two dyes.

2. Apply to wet hair in sections, starting at the back. Wrap with plastic or a towel and leave for one to six hours. This is where you need someone else to answer the door and mop up the drips for you, which will stain!

3. Rinse thoroughly and wash out all the dyestuff. Throw away any leftover mix of dye, which will not keep. After a day or two the indigo will oxidise and the hair colour will settle into a deep bluey black. That's what I'm told, anyway.

Two step method
(After reading about the whole process and preparing thoroughly to avoid spills, stains and upset.)

1. Henna your hair first, using the first method described. Mix the indigo powder with warm water and allow to sit for 10–15 minutes. This will appear green at first and be smelly. After a while it will turn blue.

2. Apply the indigo paste all over the hair as evenly as possible and wipe any drips off the skin immediately. Cover with plastic as above and leave for at least 30 minutes.

3. Rinse thoroughly and clean the bathroom!

Optional extra: Add salt (1 tsp per 100 g/3$\frac{1}{2}$ oz of indigo powder) to darken the indigo and help it cling better to the hair strand.

HAIR-CONDITIONING TREATMENTS

Hair that is out of condition usually means that your body needs help. Of course, the best way to help yourself is to eat a balanced diet, rich in fresh fruit and vegetables, which will provide all the vitamins, minerals and fatty acids that are important to maintain the health and of hair and skin. If not, maybe one of these natural treatments will give your hair a boost.

Honey
This sounds a bit messy to me, although I don't usually need to condition my hair. Mix 110 ml (4 fl oz) honey with 2 tablespoons of olive oil. Massage into the scalp well then put on a shower cap or wrap in a warm towel for 30 minutes. You could combine this with a relaxing bath.

Rosemary and honey
As an extra treat, add 4 drops of essential oil of rosemary to the honey treatment above.

Eclipta alba oil
Massaging the scalp with Eclipta alba oil helps in making hair lustrous and can also darken the hair.

Jasmine, honey and egg conditioner
This sounds best for short hair, otherwise it would take ages to get the egg and honey out. Yuck!

Warm 2 tablespoons of jojoba oil and add the egg yolk. Don't use it straight from the fridge though — let it warm up a bit first. Add 2 tablespoons of honey and a drop of jasmine oil. Apply to damp hair and leave for at least half an hour in a warm room or bath. Wash out well afterwards.

Coconut oil

Coconut oil is considered the best oil in India and has been successfully used for centuries. You could use the oil with herbs to massage the scalp prior to washing. See the face section for herbal oils.

EGGY HAIR TREATMENT

This is suggested for dry, naturally frizzy or curly locks.

Ingredients

- 115 g (4 oz) mayonnaise
- 1 egg yolk
- 1 tablespoon jojoba oil
- 5 drops grapefruit essential oil
- 2 drops patchouli essential oil

Method

Stir the mayonnaise with the egg yolk and add the jojoba oil. Mix thoroughly and then add the essential oils. After washing, apply the mix to damp hair, ensuring coverage to the very tips. Massage in, cover and leave for at least 30 minutes. Rinse out thoroughly. Well, you wouldn't want to go out with mayonnaise in your hair, would you?

OTHER PROBLEM HAIR SUGGESTIONS

Hair gel
Aloe vera gel makes a natural setting gel that won't damage your hair. This works especially well on curly hair that needs a bit of smoothing and taming.

Lemon-lime spray for wispy hair
Mix 8 tablespoons of water with 1 teaspoon of lemon juice and $1/4$ teaspoon of lime juice in a spray bottle. Shake the bottle to mix thoroughly and spray on to dry hair to tame fly away strands. Keep in the fridge.

Setting lotion
For those who still use rollers or have limp hair which quickly drops its set, you can make a setting lotion by straining the juice of a lemon with a teaspoon of vodka and 2 teaspoons of herbal infusion, such as rosemary (see below) for dark hair or chamomile for fair hair.

HAIR RINSES

Nettle (especially for fair hair)
Wash and dry nettle roots. Soak 2 handfuls of roots in 2 litres (4 pints) of cold water overnight. Bring to the boil and simmer for 10–15 minutes. Strain and use the liquid as a hair rinse.

Honey
Stir a teaspoon of honey into 1 litre (2 pints) of warm water. After shampooing and rinsing, pour the mixture through your hair. Do not rinse out.

Vinegar
Used as a hair rinse, vinegar neutralises the alkali left by shampoos. It will give your hair an all out shine,

and remove surplus soap. Add a tablespoon or two of vinegar to the final rinse. The smell doesn't linger.

When you have dyed your hair, rinse with warm water then dilute white vinegar with water for the final rinse. Use the water as cold as you can stand. This seals your colour so it doesn't fade out as quickly.

Lemon (for fair hair)
After shampooing, treat your hair with a final rinse of water and lemon juice (half a lemon mixed with 500 ml/17 fl oz of water) to fight dandruff and sweep the soap film and excess oils. This might make a nice change from vinegar and smells a bit better.

Chamomile tea (for fair hair)
Create natural highlights by making an infusion of chamomile flowers in hot water. When cool use this as a rinse.

HAIR LIGHTENERS

Hair can be lightened or highlighted with lemon juice in a solution with water. Make sure that you have equal quantities, or slightly more lemon juice. Comb through and leave for a while before washing as normal. Lemon, unfortunately isn't very good for your hair, so don't overdo it.

Blonder blondes
Lemon juice applied to the hair is a natural lightener. A suggestion for blondes who want to be blonder is to mix the juice of one lemon or two limes with some mild shampoo. Massage in and sit in the sun for 20 minutes before rinsing and conditioning, as the juice won't do your hair any favours.

DANDRUFF TREATMENTS

Some of these suggestions might be worth a try.
Heat coconut oil with 20 g (1 oz) of neem extract
powder and apply to your hair once a week.
Presumably, wash with a mild shampoo afterwards:

- ○ Mix 1 teaspoon lemon juice with 2 teaspoons
  vinegar and massage onto the scalp. Follow this up
  with a mild shampoo or an egg shampoo.
- ○ Mix 100 ml (3½ fl oz) witch hazel with 1 tablespoon
  fresh lemon juice in 200 ml (7 fl oz) water.
  Shampoo your hair and apply to the scalp when
  the hair is still wet. Repeat several times until the
  dandruff is treated.
- ○ As a hair wash for treatment against dandruff, use
  the water cooled from boiling up beetroot to rinse
  the hair and scalp. The Victorians used this for a
  light colouring rinse.

HAIR LOSS AND CIDER VINEGAR

Although we lose hair daily that is replaced, greater
hair loss is primarily due to a tissue salt deficiency, so
cider vinegar with its 'wonder products' will re-
establish a natural balance, and supply the deficiencies
where needed. By taking cider vinegar treatment the
hair will maintain its natural growth. This will take
approximately two months, so persevere. The dosage is
1 teaspoon of cider vinegar to a glass of water to be
taken with or between meals.

SHAMPOOS

Dry bicarb shampoo

I remember someone at school doing this with talcum powder when I was a teenager and everyone was obsessed with not having greasy hair. I can't think of when there isn't time to wash your hair nowadays in the shower, apart from when camping and/or faced with a lack of water. However, the tip is: sprinkle bicarbonate of soda on to your hair and rub through. Comb out and dry in warm air. Luckily I don't have greasy hair anymore!

Dry oatmeal shampoo

This sounds even less pleasant. Sprinkle 1 teaspoon each of oatmeal and bicarbonate of soda on your head. Massage in for a few minutes, then comb or brush out. Again, warm air will help to get rid of residue.

Rosemary shampoo

Adding fresh herbs to ready made unscented shampoo creates a refreshing, stimulating shampoo that may also help hair growth and darken hair colour. Take a good bunch of fresh rosemary and bring 225 ml (8 fl oz) water to the boil. Add the herbs and simmer for 15–20 minutes. Strain well and add the liquid to 115 ml (4 fl oz) unscented liquid soap. Add a few drops of rosemary oil and mix well. This can be kept in a labelled plastic bottle as required.

Herbal shampoo

For a truly different experience, make a paste of extracts of shikakai, soapnut and amla powder. Use this as you would shampoo.

Fuller's earth shampoo

Mix an equal quantity of Fuller's earth with dried orris root powder. Part the hair and sprinkle in the mixture. Don't rub it into the scalp. Cover and leave for 5 minutes before brushing vigorously with a towel round your shoulders.

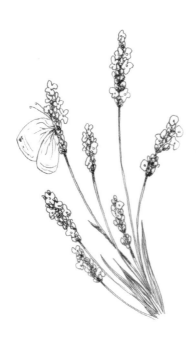

BATH-TIME TREATMENTS

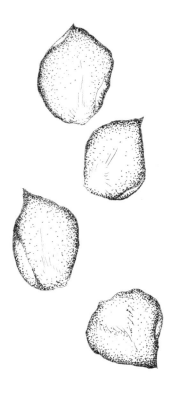

BATH-TIME TREATMENTS

Baths can be used to help a wide range of ailments and to help you relax. If you can't run away to a spa or afford a pricey treatment, try one of these. Don't fill the bath too fully so that you can add more hot water when required. It will revive you in no time.

SOOTHING SOAKS

AROMATIC BATHS FOR ALL REQUIREMENTS

Dilute 10 drops of essential oils in 3 tablespoons of honey or 225 ml (8 fl oz) of milk and pour the mixture in the tub filled with water.

For relaxation add:	Lavender
	Geranium
	Sandalwood
	Chamomile
	Frankincense
For a detox effect choose:	Rosemary
	Geranium
	Juniper
	Lemon oil
For stress use:	Lavender
	Basil
	Geranium
If you have a cold try:	Eucalyptus
	Camphor
	Sage
	Pine
	Thyme

HERBAL BATHS

You could use one of the many spare washing powder bags around the house for this. Put the chosen herbs in a small mesh bag or piece of muslin. Let it steep in the bath for a few minutes. You can use the bag to gently scrub the body.

For a rejuvenating bath use equal parts of:
> Yarrow flowers
> Elder flowers
> Mint leaves
> Rose petals

For a soothing bath that also increases circulation choose:
> Comfrey and mint leaves
> Chamomile
> Lavender

SEA SALT BATH SOAK

Sea salt can be used for a hot soak. Try adding a cup of sea salt to a bath and soaking for at least ten minutes. You will feel soothed and clean. Add a few drops of your favourite scented oils to soften the skin.

BICARB AND SEA SALT DETOX

Use one part (3 tablespoons) bicarbonate of soda to one part sea salt in a hot bath. Lie back and relax for 20 minutes. Rinse off or shower to remove the salt. For a more luxurious soak, add a tablespoon of citric acid and a few drops of essential oil to the salt and bicarbonate of soda.

You can mix up a jar full and add food colouring as well for a gift idea.

SCENTED BATH SALTS

> 200 g (7 oz) coarse sea salt
> 1 tablespoon cornflour
> 50 g (1³/4 oz) Epsom salts

Plus either:

> few drops rose oil
>
> 1 tablespoon dried rose petals
>
> 1 tablespoon dried peony petals

or

> few drops lemon or orange oil
>
> 1 tablespoon calendula petals
>
> 1 teaspoon safflower

Method

Place the sea salts, cornflour and Epsom salts into a mixing bowl. Add the oil and blend well. Place in an airtight container with the dried flowers of your choice until required. Use a handful of the mix in a bath of hot water.

OIL-FREE OATMEAL BATH SOAK

Ingredients

> 115 g (4 oz) oatmeal
>
> 115 g (4 oz) cornflour

Method

This mix can cause havoc with drains, so put the ingredients into the foot from an old pair of tights so that you can remove it from the bath and discard in the bin. It will save a lot of cleaning of plugholes!

CINNAMON OATMEAL MILK BATH

Ingredients

> 115 g (4 oz) corn flour
>
> 225 g (8 oz) powdered milk
>
> 50 g (2 oz) medium oatmeal
>
> $1/2$ teaspoon cinnamon

This is enough for 4–5 baths and can be stored in a jar or decorative container

Method
Mix all ingredients in blender or food processor until you have a fine powder. Add about 2 tablespoons of the mixture to the water for a soothing bath.

SIMPLE OATMEAL BATH SOAK

This is good for a dry, itchy skin. The other foot from the old tights will make it less messy and easier to manage.

Ingredients
> 3 tablespoons olive oil
> 5 drops essential oil of your choice (optional)
> 2 to 3 cups porridge oatflakes (not instant)

Method
Combine the essential oils for an hour or two with the olive oil before starting. Mix in the oats until they are coated with the oils. Pour into the old tights and tie up securely.

Add to a warm bath and soak yourself for at least 20 minutes. Dispose of the bag immediately after use.

SPORT RELIEF SOAK

Mmm, smell that wintergreen...

> 1 cup coarse sea salt
> 2 drops of wintergreen essential oil
> 2 drops of eucalyptus essential oil
> 1 drop of peppermint essential oil

Just add all the ingredients together and mix well.

SKIN SOFTENING HONEY BATH

For a classically simple treat, try adding three or four tablespoons of honey to the bath water. You will enjoy a silky, fragrant bath.

FOAMING HONEY BATH
(enough for 4 baths)

Ingredients
- 225 ml (8 fl oz) sweet almond oil, light olive or sesame oil
- 175 g (6 oz) honey
- 115 g (4 oz) liquid soap
- 1 tablespoon vanilla extract

Method
Put the oil into a medium bowl and carefully stir in remaining ingredients until fully blended. Pour into a clean plastic bottle with a lid and a label. Shake gently before using.

Pour into running water and enjoy a warm, silky escape.

LAVENDER AND HONEY MILK BATH
(for two baths)

Ingredients
- 3 tablespoons dried lavender flowers
- 350 ml (12 fl oz) whole milk or cream
- 115 g (4 oz) honey

Method
The lavender can be gathered from the garden after flowering on a dry day. The easiest way is to hang the flower heads upside down in a paper bag and hang in

a dry place. As the seed ripen they will be contained in the bag and you won't end up with lavender all over the place.

You can process the lavender flowers in a blender until they become a powder, or grind them in a mortar and pestle. Whisk together this lavender powder and the milk and honey, then pour into a jar and seal. Before use, shake the jar and pour half of the mixture into a running bath. Store covered in the refrigerator for up to a week.

HERBAL BATH VINEGAR

Mix lavender, lady's mantle leaves and rose petals with cider vinegar and allow to sit for 2–4 weeks. You can use this as a facial tonic or as a bath additive.

SUGAR AND SPICE TREAT

Mix together 4 tablespoons of bicarbonate of soda, 2 of sugar, 1 teaspoon of ground cinnamon, a pinch of ground ginger and a pinch of ground cloves. This will keep for some time. When you are ready for a bath, take 2 tablespoons of the dry mix and add to running water.

BATH BOMBS

Did you know that the main ingredient in fizzy bath products is bicarbonate of soda? You can make your own with three parts bicarbonate of soda to one part citric acid. Add your own fragrance oils or colouring. You can buy moulds for this purpose, but I think egg boxes would work just as well.

Mix together the dry ingredients and add water-based

colour (not pigment, as this may stain). Don't be tempted to overdo the colour as this will be stronger when mixed with water. Mix with the oil of your choice (lavender is good for relaxation) until it clumps together in your hand. If the mixture is too stiff, add a little base oil, like almond oil. Put small balls of this into the egg box to dry. This will take a day or two. When you want to use one, just put in a bath of water and enjoy.

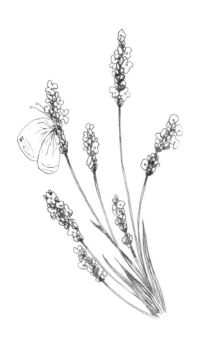

HOME-MADE SOAP

I have included the following for interest, although there are quite a lot of ingredients involved. You can purchase soap base quite cheaply by mail order or online if you have trouble finding it locally.

HERBAL OATMEAL SOAP

This herbal, aromatic and soothing soap is great for dry skin. The recipe will make several bars. You can add or change the herbs and dried flowers to suit your preferences.

Ingredients

350 ml (12 fl oz) distilled water

85 g (3 oz) oatmeal

500 g (1 lb) soap base

1/4 teaspoon rosemary essential oil

1/4 teaspoon sage essential oil

1/4 teaspoon lavender essential oil

4 tablespoons dried chamomile flowers

4 tablespoons calendula petals

2 tablespoons dried nettle

2 tablespoons dried rosemary

2 tablespoons dried rose hips

Method

A few hours before making this soap, combine the water, oatmeal and herbs in a saucepan. Heat to boiling, then cover and simmer for at least 30 minutes. Cool, preferably covered.

Strain through a double or triple muslin cloth or pair of tights, saving the liquid. Throw away the oatmeal and herbs.

Cut the soap base into small cubes and place in a microwave-safe measuring jug/bowl. Either microwave on a high setting for 30 seconds at a time, stirring in-between until the base is nearly melted, or melt the soap in a container in a pan of water on the cooker.

Stir the base slowly to avoid air bubbles. Your now-liquid base will be very hot. Let it cool down until you can comfortably touch it, stirring slowly. Add the herbal liquid and essential oils. Stir gently and pour into moulds or small clean containers that you can get the soap out of when set.The bars can be used as soon as they are completely hardened. Use for face and body in bath or shower.

CREAMY OATMEAL SOAP

Ingredients
    500 g (1 lb) soap base
    $\frac{1}{2}$ teaspoon fragrance oil of your choice
    4 tablespoons oatmeal

Method
Melt the soap in a microwave or double boiler until fully melted. Do not let it get too hot. Allow to cool slightly until it forms a thin skin on the top.

Quickly add the fragrance and stir slightly. Don't stir too much as this will cause air bubbles to form and the soap will cool too fast.

When the soap starts to thicken to a porridge consistency, add the oats and stir gently. If the soap is too runny, all the oats will end up on one side. Pour into moulds or small containers to cool.

INVIGORATING SCRUBS

SALT AND LEMON MASSAGE

Mix 30 g (1½ oz) of hard sea salt with 12 drops of lemon essential oil and enough warm water to make an even paste. Put on a massage glove and start massaging your body with the mixture. Pay special attention to your thighs, backside and stomach. Shower off afterwards.

CHOCOLATE HONEY SCRUB

The original recipe calls for 225 g (8 oz) salt, which seems rather excessive so I have left this ingredient out. Come to think of it, the whole recipe now sounds a bit bizarre.

Ingredients
>   3 tablespoons cocoa powder
>   225 ml (8 fl oz) honey
>   50 ml (2 fl oz) oil

Method
Mix the honey and oil together and stir in the cocoa. Gently massage all over before rinsing in the shower or bath.

MORNING BODY SCRUB

Ingredients
>   50 g (2 oz) freshly ground coffee
>   50 ml (2 fl oz) skimmed milk
>   2 tablespoons wheat germ
>   2 tablespoons honey
>   1 tablespoon grape seed or light oil
>   1 egg white

Method

Mix together the milk, honey, oil and egg white.
Slowly add the coffee and wheat germ, avoiding
lumps. The scrub should be even with a slightly gritty
texture. Allow to stand. Apply all over in the shower
or bath, using a body sponge to aid in exfoliation.
Rinse off and dry. Apply your favourite moisturiser.
Any remaining scrub can be kept for a day or two.

ROSEMARY BODY SCRUB
Very thorough, for real toughies

115 g (4 oz) coarse sea salt
4 tablespoons rosemary oil

Put some oil on a loofah then dip it into the salt.
Using circular movements, rub over the skin. Give
extra attention to rough areas. Continue to do this
until your body is covered. Rinse with a warm water
shower and pat dry. Follow up with moisturiser.

COFFEE AND GRAPEFRUIT THIGH SCRUB

This makes 2 applications, if you can bear it! It will
keep in an airtight container until you forget what it
was like the first time. Coffee stimulates fatty
congestion and grapefruit stimulates the lymphatic
system, removing toxins from the body.

115 g (4 oz) sea salt
4 tablespoons clay
1 teaspoon ground coffee
1 teaspoon of cinnamon
10 drops peppermint oil
15 drops grapefruit essential oil
15 drops orange essential oil

Method

Combine all the ingredients together, breaking up any clumps. To use mix 2 tablespoons of the mix with enough water or milk to form a smooth paste. Massage into the thigh and buttock areas. Rinse off in the shower.

MASSAGE OIL

Add 5–10 drops ginger oil to 25 ml (1 fl oz) almond oil for rheumatism or lumbago. You could also use juniper or eucalyptus oil instead of almond oil.

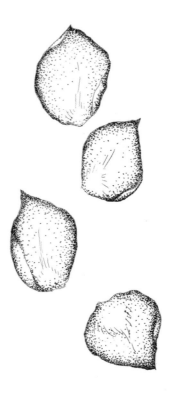

GLOSSARY

This section may help to explain some of the scientific names and terms used when talking about cosmetics. I have also included some everyday ingredients that are not 'natural' and which you may wish to avoid.

Alpha hydroxy acids (AHAs)
AHAs were introduced in the 1990s. Derived from fruit and milk sugars, they are weak hygroscopic acids (see below) and can be synthetic or naturally occurring. Originally called fruit acids, they have been used in many skincare products. Such products claim to reduce fine lines, smooth and give a firmer feel to the skin. They are said to promote production of collagen and elastin as well (see below). They only work superficially on younger skin, so all the hype about reducing wrinkles doesn't apply to young skin which doesn't have wrinkles anyway. They can give protection through moisturising and a feel good factor, although the cost might make you less enthusiastic, given that you could use real fruit for the same effects. They are not an anti-ageing remedy but are safe when used in moderation. AHAs are sometimes present in chemical peels and they can cause mild irritation and flaking or blistering. They can also increase sensitivity to the sun. Some important AHAs are glycolic acid and lactic acid (see below). Others such malic acid, from apples and pears, and tartaric acid, from fermented grapes, are still being investigated. Citric acid comes, unsurprisingly, from citrus fruits. Alpha hydroxy acids found in skin-care products work best in a concentration of 5 per cent to 8 per cent and at a pH of around 3.0. They require daily application over several months to be effective.

Antioxidants
See Free radicals

Betacarotene
The vitamin A that is found in colourful fruits and vegetables such as beetroot and carrots, contains betacarotene, which, once eaten, converts into vitamin A. While excessive amounts of vitamin A in supplement form can be toxic, the body will only convert as much vitamin A from betacarotene as it needs.

Ceramides
Ceramides make up most of the fat layer that holds the skin cells together in a firm, smooth structure. They maintain moisture

retention and provide hydration, along with cholesterol and free fatty acids. Ceramides account for about half of this layer. The water content of healthy skin, normally between 10 per cent and 20 per cent, is dependent on ceramides. Below 10 per cent the skin will be dry. Synthetic ceramides became commercially available in the 1990s and have been shown to reduce some cases of dermatitis. There are several types that claim to visibly reverse the signs of ageing by increasing the thickness of the epidermis, improving texture and plumping out the skin. The use of some chemicals, such as detergents like sodium laurel sulphate, speeds up the loss of water and may take some time to readjust.

Citric acid
Citric acid is widely used in the cosmetics industry and is another AHA. It is used as a preservative and to regulate pH balance. It also has antioxidant properties and is a good toner.

Collagen
Collagen is a protein found in skin, bone, cartilage and other connective tissues. It forms the main structural component of the lower layer of the skin or dermis. It accounts for the strength of the skin and is produced by cells called fibroblasts. Along with elastin it provides structure and firmness to body tissues. As we get older changes prevent proteins working effectively, so we lose some of that firmness and eventually acquire wrinkles instead. Reduction of collagen breakdown is said to be achievable by stimulating collagen production and, in so doing, reduce wrinkles and improve skin texture. Vitamin C is important for synthesis of collagen and is also an antioxidant. Unfortunately you can't just take large quantities of vitamin C to prevent ageing because it cannot be stored. What is more, you might do yourself more harm than good.

Cytophylactic
A plant is said to be cytophylactic if it helps to heal skin or regenerate cells. Some examples are eucalyptus, centella or Indian pennywort, lavender and orange.

Demulcent
A demulcent is something that forms a soothing film over a mucous membrane such as the throat, relieving minor pain and inflammation. Glycerine and honey are good examples of materials that have cosmetic uses as well. Quercetin, part of the pigment

also found in the skins of apples and red onions, is a powerful antioxidant, natural antihistamine and anti-inflammatory. Gum made from pieces of plants dissolved in water is a demulcent and protects inflamed surfaces.

Dermis
This is the second layer under the epidermis that is made of connective tissue: collagen, elastic and reticular fibres. The dermis protects the body from strain and stress. It is this layer that houses nerve endings, hair follicles, blood vessels and several glands. These are eccrine (sweat) glands, sebaceous (oil) glands and apocrine glands (scent). The blood vessels provide oxygen to the dermis as well as to the stratum basale and also take away waste matter. The dermis varies in thickness from 0.3 mm to 3 mm. Nerve endings supply information to the brain on pain, temperature, itchiness and other sensations.

Elastin
Elastin is a protein found in skin and body tissue. It helps to keep skin both flexible and tight. It also helps to keep skin smooth as it stretches during normal activities like flexing muscles, talking or eating, or during pregnancy when the skin is required to stretch a great deal. Elastin diminishes naturally as we get older. Any elastin listed as an ingredient in anti-ageing products does not come from human sources, but from animal sources such as cows and birds. Nice! Elastin in skin care products does not penetrate the skin layer, so cannot be effective.

Emollients
These are substances that soften and soothe the skin. Examples of natural emollients are almond oil, cocoa butter and egg. They are used to correct dryness and scaly skin. They are a key component in the manufacture of lipstick, lotions and other cosmetic products.

Epidermis
The epidermis or outer layer is divided into five sublayers. The thickness varies from 0.05 mm on the eyelids to 1.5 mm on the soles of your feet. Cells grow from deep layers and migrate outwards to form a protective barrier of dead cells at the surface, called the stratum corneum. This multi-layered structure consists of layers of fats and both water-loving (hydrophilic) and water-hating (hydrophobic) areas. This creates an efficient barrier against chemicals that are insoluble in fat and against those that are

insoluble in water. Overcoming this barrier is a challenge for the development of drugs delivered through the skin such as nicotine, pain relief or HRT patches.

Below this top layer is the stratum lucidum. This is only present in the thick, hairless skin of the palm of hand and the soles of the feet. Three more layers below this make up the rest of the epidermis. The deepest layer is called the stratum germinativum or stratum basale, where the cells are shaped like columns. Here the cells divide and push previously formed cells up into higher layers. As the cells move into the higher layers, they flatten and eventually die. This is the part of the skin where melanin is produced from melanocyte cells.

Essential oils
Essential oils are natural substances derived from shrubs and trees, flowers, leaves and grasses. They are obtained through pressing or distillation. Some oils such as citrus oils are cheaper to produce than other oils because the trees and fruits grow quite easily in the right climate. There is a large amount of oil present in the peel that can be extracted by cold pressing or by distillation. Lemon oil, oleum limonis, is especially easy to obtain.

Essential oils were discovered as having antiseptic properties during outbreaks of cholera in France in the nineteenth century, when workers in perfume factories showed greater immunity to the disease, although they have been used since Egyptian times to protect the skin. See the history section. The addition of a few drops of essential oil offers not only fragrance to a product but also several therapeutic properties and mean that synthetic additives are not needed to preserve a mix. For example, zingiberene is the predominant constituent of the oil of ginger, accounting for 20 per cent to 30 per cent of the volatile oil. It functions as an insecticide or repellent while zingiberol is an alcohol with the fragrance of ginger. Their effects can benefit skin and hair and can last from hours to days. If they are too concentrated they can cause skin rashes.

Fatty acids
Fatty acids are a part of the lipid layer, and help maintain the suppleness and elasticity of skin. Their deficiency results in loss of moisture and hardening and drying of the skin. Along with ceramides, oxidants, AHAs and vitamins A and E, they work to nourish from deep within. See also palmitic acid, stearic acid and oleic acid.

Free radicals and antioxidants
Free radicals cause damage to cells by attacking molecules for their electrons. Once damaged, a molecule becomes a free radical itself. Antioxidants neutralise free radicals by donating one of their own electrons, without becoming unstable themselves. Instead, they act as scavengers, cleaning up and helping to prevent cell damage that could lead to disease. Some free radicals arise normally, when the body's immune system's cells purposefully create them to neutralise viruses and bacteria.

Environmental factors such as pollution, radiation, cigarette smoke and herbicides, can also create free radicals. It is important to note that free radical damage intensifies as we get older, so eating foods high in vitamin C and E and also those high in fibre can only do good. Ingredients containing vitamins A, C and E help the body to resist free radicals that prematurely age the skin. They interrupt oxidation, the spoilage process that makes skin collagen break down.

Glycolic acid is the most widely used and most effective AHA and is manufactured from sugar cane. It is used to exfoliate and moisturise. The percentage concentrate of glycolic acid in a product seems to be around 10 per cent, which some people deem too low to be effective, but concentration levels of glycolic acid in some chemical peels can be as high as 50 per cent or more. This level of exfoliation works under the top layers of dead skin and peels off the layers, promoting the growth of new skin. After a chemical peel the skin will look extremely sunburnt, so several days of recovery are often necessary. Glycolic acid is often combined with other AHAs that promote more moisturisers and neutralisers. This is not something to do just before a big occasion, when you want to look your best!

Humectant
A humectant is a material that increases the water-holding capacity of the skin. Examples are glycerine, honey and lactic acid.

Hygroscopic substances
Hygroscopic material attracts moisture from the atmosphere, so any substance that can be added to the skin or hair to retain moisture falls into this category. Examples are glycerine, honey and aloe vera.

Lactic acid
Lactic acid is an AHA. Cleopatra didn't know she was using a mild AHA when she bathed in sour goats milk, I bet. It is less irritating

than glycolic acid, and has good hydrating properties, so it is beneficial for those who have sensitive skin.

Linoleic acid

Linoleic acid is a fatty acid used in cosmetics as an emollient, antioxidant and cell regulator, also considered to promote healthy skin growth. It is also an anti-inflammatory agent and can be found in blackcurrant oil, evening primrose oil and borage.

Liposomes

Liposomes are made from fatty substances and create tiny bubbles made out of material very similar to a cell membrane. They can be used to deliver drugs to treat diseases including cancer. Cosmetically, they are used like capsules to deliver active ingredients to the epidermis and dermis. Washing out of the beneficial action of these substances, for example in sunscreen products, is slowed down. When a cosmetic containing liposomes is applied to the skin, the liposomes left on the skin begin to merge with the cellular membranes, allowing for very exact delivery of materials to cells over a long period.

Melanin

Melanin is a skin pigment that gives the skin its colour. Dark-skinned people have more melanin than light-skinned people. Melanin acts as a sunscreen and protects the skin from ultraviolet light, which is why fairer skinned people are more susceptible to sunburn. Melanin is also found in hair, tissue, the iris and other areas of the body. Freckles are small concentrated areas where melanin production has increased. Melanin is produced by cells called melanocytes, found in the stratum basale. These cells increase production in response to exposure to the sun, giving rise to browning of the skin. Lack of melanin gives rise to albinism.

Moisturiser

Any material that adds moisture to the skin can be termed a moisturiser, but the word is usually used for a finished product. Emollient is often substituted, but this means softener rather than adding moisture. Naturally moisturising ingredients include oil of apricot, coconut, safflower, sesame, soya bean, almond and jojoba. Jojoba wax, lanolin and shea butter are other examples.

Oleic acid

Oleic acid is a monounsaturated omega-9 fatty acid found in animal and vegetable sources, and is also present in cocoa butter. A main

source of this acid is olive oil, used for centuries in the
Mediterranean. Grape seed oil also contains high levels.
Oleic acid is often used to make soap and is present in a
number of cosmetics as a moisturising agent.

Oleoresin

An oleoresin is a mixture of oil containing turpentine and a resin.
Now before we all get the wrong idea and get confused with
solvents and paint strippers, we are talking medically here.
Turpentine was originally distilled from pine trees and particularly
from the terebinth tree. You may or may not be interested to know
that turpentine is a highly effective treatment for lice. Some
modern products still contain it. It is not normally taken internally
today. Oleoresin is extracted from plants such as capsicums (or
peppers) and ginger. The oil holds the resins in solution.

Palmitic acid

Palmitic acid is one of the most common saturated fatty acids
found in animals and plants. It is a major component of the oil
from coconut palm trees. Butter, cheese, milk, cocoa butter and
meat also contain this fatty acid. It is used in soaps and cosmetics,
as well as being a food additive. The detergent effect that creates
foam can cause drying.

Parabens

Parabens are chemicals widely used as preservatives in the cosmetic
and pharmaceutical industries, primarily for their fungicidal
properties. They are commonly found in shampoos, moisturisers,
shaving gels, cleansers, spray tanning solution and toothpaste. They
are also used as food additives, being cheap to produce. Their long
use is now being questioned. For most individuals parabens do not
cause a problem, but those with sensitive skin may suffer skin
irritation, dermatitis and allergic reactions.

Retinol and retinoids

Retinoids are vitamin A compounds, which are found in animal
sources such as liver, kidney, eggs and dairy produce, whereas
carotenoids are found in plants. Retinol is one of these animal
compounds. Retinol is a component in some anti-ageing creams but
some claim that it leaves the skin more sensitive to sunlight and
that some people are very sensitive to its use, resulting in very dry,
flaky skin. Skin cells have specialised enzymes that convert various
forms of vitamin A into retinoic acid under certain conditions,
although in small quantities. Most creams containing retinol don't

contain enough to make a difference. Higher concentrations are too irritating to the skin. Also, retinol is fairly unstable and its effectiveness is lost in storage.

Saponin
Saponins come from plants and dissolve in water to create a soapy froth. Sapon actually means 'soap'. They are mild detergents used commercially and are also useful for astringent and cleansing action. Saponins are for external consumption only and can be poisonous.

Skin
We talk about skincare and either lavish products on it all our lives or abuse it with harsh chemicals, but how much do you know about your skin? Skin is soft, pliable, strong, waterproof and self-repairing. Without it you would be a mess. It is the largest single organ in your body and works like a protective wrapper. With the layer of fat underneath, it insulates and protects, keeps germs out and fluids in. Skin functions in the following ways:
• protects from infection, disease and a hostile environment
• maintains proper temperature
• gathers sensory information.
Adults have nearly 2 square metres of skin, which is being regenerated all the time. You are likely to shed some 18 kg (40 lbs) of skin in a lifetime. Every minute 30,000–40,000 dead skin cells fall from your body. Every four weeks, children's bodies make a whole new layer of skin cells. We shed the top layer about every two weeks. Human skin is organised into distinct layers; the epidermis, dermis and subcutaneous tissue.

Skin damage from UV rays
Research into nutrition has discovered that various foods improve the resilience of your skin against UV damage. This reduces your risk of sunburn and various skin cancers. Thirteen nutrients have been identified that increase the skin's protection. Ten of these are found in spinach and chard, so eating green leafy vegetables will really help your skin. Betacarotene, which is present in leafy vegetables such as spinach, has been studied in connection with the incidence of skin cancer in Australia. In population surveys among men, researchers found that those who ate more foods rich in betacarotene had a lower statistical risk of developing skin cancer.

Sodium lauryl sulphate
This synthetic chemical is widely used in shampoos for its detergent and foam producing properties. It is also found in soaps, toothpaste,

bubble baths and shaving foams. Industrially, it is used to degrease engines, clean floors and wash cars, so we are talking strong stuff here. It is cheap and effective at cleaning up grease, but not the sort of treatment you want to put your hair through very often. It can cause eye irritations, skin rashes, scurf and allergic reactions.

Stearalkonium chloride
This chemical is used in hair conditioners and creams. It was developed as an industrial fabric softener and is cheaper to produce than protein and herbal hair products. It makes hair shinier and easier to comb and reduces static. The stearic acid (see below) used to make it can be found in natural fats, but the synthetic substance is believed to damage hair and even be toxic. You can achieve shiny hair with lots of other natural rinses.

Stearic acid
This pearly or waxy fatty acid substance is found in cocoa butter, but is also produced from animal fats and other vegetable sources. Small flakes can be used as an emulsifying agent in creams, lotions and deodorants.

Subcutaneous tissue
This is the third and lowest of the three layers of skin. The subcutaneous layer contains fat and connective tissue and larger blood vessels and nerves. It lies between the dermis and muscles. This layer is important in the regulation of temperature of the skin and of the whole body. The actual thickness varies throughout the body and from person to person.

Surfactants
This word was coined in the 1950s from surface active agent. Surfactants act as wetting agents and also degrease and emulsify oils and fats. They are used in washing powders to suspend and remove dirt. Surfactants are also used in most forms of cleansers. Many are considered gentle and effective for most skin types but some types can be drying and irritating for the skin.

Vitamin A
Vitamin A is a group of compounds that play an important role in vision, bone growth, reproduction and cell growth. It helps to regulate the immune system, preventing or fighting off infections by making white blood cells that destroy harmful bacteria and viruses. Vitamin A promotes healthy surface linings to the eyes, respiratory, urinary and intestinal tracts. When those linings break

down, it becomes easier for bacteria to enter the body and cause infection. Vitamin A also helps the skin and mucous membranes function as a barrier to bacteria and viruses. See also betacarotene and retinoids.

Vitamin B_2 (Riboflavin)

Riboflavin has a number of important functions. It helps keep skin, eyes, the nervous system and mucous membranes healthy. It may help the body absorb iron from the food we eat and it helps produce steroids and red blood cells.

Vitamin B_5 (pantothenic acid)

This important vitamin is the key to metabolism of carbohydrates, fats and proteins. In combination with zinc, it is claimed that B_5 can prevent hair from turning grey in rats. It can promote resistance to the stress of cold immersion and may be tied to tumour inhibition. In combination with vitamin C it maintains capillary walls and promotes circulation. It is also said to be antibacterial and promote pain relief.

Vitamin C

Vitamin C is the main water-soluble antioxidant in the body and is vital for the healthy functioning of the immune system. It is good at preventing common colds and may also help to reduce recurrent ear infections. It is essential for healthy teeth and gums, helps wounds heal, helps fractures to mend and heals scar tissue. Deficiency led to scurvy among sailors in the past. Vitamin C helps vitamin E become active. It is particularly effective in combating free-radical formation caused by pollution and cigarette smoke. Vitamin C has been shown to help slow the production of age spots and to provide some UV protection.

Vitamin E

Vitamin E is the body's main fat-soluble antioxidant. It plays a big role in preventing cardiovascular disease and is one of the main antioxidants found in cholesterol. It helps prevent free radicals that would damage the cell membranes by oxidizing the cholesterol. If cholesterol is oxidized it causes problems by sticking to blood vessel walls and blocking arteries. Vitamin E oil is obtained by vacuum distillation of vegetable fats. Recent studies have suggested that Vitamin E oil may retard ageing.